Why do you overeat?
When all you want is to be slim

The Harcombe Diet®

Published by Columbus Publishing Ltd 2013
www.columbuspublishing.co.uk

ISBN 978-1-907797-24-8

A CIP record of this book is available from the British Library.

Cover design by Lewis Kokoc & Andy Harcombe

The content of this book is intended to inform, entertain and provoke your
thinking. This is not intended as medical advice. It may, however, make you
question current medical and nutritional advice. That's your choice. It's your
life and health in your hands. Neither the author nor the publisher can be held
responsible or liable for any loss or claim arising from the use, or misuse, of
the content of this book.

COLUMBUS PUBLISHING

Thank You...

Thank you to the growing number of fans of The Harcombe Diet for trusting nature to feed you better than 'food' manufacturers. Thank you for spreading the word and for encouraging others to eat real food. All your weight loss and better health stories have made what we do so worth-while.

Thank you to Harcombe Diet experts Kate, Peggy & Priscilla for your meticulous checking of the final manuscript.

Thank you Andy for everything that you are and do.

Dedication...

This book is dedicated to Earl Lynch, without whom none of this would have happened!

To find out more...

www.zoeharcombe.com

www.theharcombediet.com

www.theharcombedietclub.com

www.theobesityepidemic.org

Contents

Why do you overeat?
When all you want is to be slim

The Harcombe Diet®

Chapter One

****

How did The Harcombe Diet come about?

This first chapter is both an introduction to and a summary of the whole book. It takes you through my journey of discovering The Harcombe Diet. In doing so, it will introduce you to three conditions that cause insatiable food cravings. All will be comprehensively explained later in the book. For now, just enjoy the story and know that you are just a short read away from having the knowledge to transform your relationship with food and, therefore, your weight.

If you currently feel addicted to food, out of control around food and overeat, despite so desperately wanting to be slim, I can promise that discovering these conditions will change your life. Here's how they changed mine...

Background

There were three key events in my life that led to me doing what I do today:

1) My interest in anything to do with food and what we eat first started when my brother, Adrian, developed type 1 diabetes – he was 15 and I was 13. I witnessed him drop 20 pounds, in as many days, right in front of my eyes. Looking back, the diagnosis took unnecessarily long – the symptoms of being a teenager, dramatic weight loss and insatiable thirst should have been so obvious, but this was years ago and we were probably less switched on to diabetes then. Before long, mum, dad and I had been called in to the hospital to have a family training session to understand the difference between Adrian being in a state of *hypo*glycaemia (low blood glucose levels) vs. *hyper*glycaemia (high blood

glucose levels). As soon as Adrian came home, I was then helping my big brother inject insulin into his body and starting to make the obvious connection between insulin, carbohydrate and weight.

The family diet also changed overnight – gone were the high teas, with scones and cake, from my parents' upbringing and in came 'meat and two veg' kind of meals; much better for the whole family.

2) I developed anorexia when I was 15. My personal view of anorexia, from experience and research since, is that – especially when developed in child or teenager years – it is a psychological condition. It is fundamentally about low self esteem and a high need to control something and food in and exercise done become things that one can, and does, control.

I now also know that, for many anorexics and for so many calorie counters who just didn't get as far as anorexia, under-eating leads to over-eating just as night follows day. When people ask me how to stop bingeing I say stop starving; when they ask how to stop starving I say stop bingeing – these are the yin and yang of dieting.

3) The final trigger event, which started my years of research into overeating, was having bulimia while studying at Cambridge University. What should have been the time of my life was being wasted bingeing on crisps, cakes, chocolate, biscuits and all sorts of junk. I asked myself the question – I'm more than half bright – why am I doing this? Why do I overeat when all I want is to be slim?

Why do you overeat? When all you want is to be slim became the title of my first book – first published in 2004. *Stop Counting Calories & Start Losing Weight* was published in 2008 as the core book for The Harcombe Diet. However, the title of this book has always been my favourite – as it is the million dollar question and the one that I spent so many years trying to answer. This book is a completely revised version of the original and it is the psychological partner to *Stop Counting*

Calories & Start Losing Weight. If you want the fullest details of The Harcombe Diet possible, 100 Q&As, recipes and why the diet ticks all the boxes, *Stop Counting Calories & Start Losing Weight* is the book for you. If you want the physical and psychological answer to the question on the cover of this book – this is it.

Why do we overeat?

When I set out to try to understand why I couldn't stop eating when I wanted more than anything to be slim, there was no internet and research was nowhere near as easy as it is now. I trotted off to book shops and libraries and looked for anything that seemed to provide a lead...

Food Intolerance

My first breakthrough was going to a great GP (General Practitioner/doctor) while I was at Cambridge. He was a young doctor and he may have been clued up on the latest thinking as a result. I had been to GP's before about feeling out of control around food and they just wanted to refer me to a counsellor. I found counsellors pretty useless to be honest. They were either too fat or too thin – so not the role models I was looking for – and none could explain why I only wanted certain foods. They all wanted to explore different psychological strands and I just wanted to get the heck out of the room, so that I could eat a box of chocolates!

This GP was different and wonderful. I took in a written list of symptoms – bloating, gaining or losing pounds literally overnight, insatiable cravings, mood swings, energy highs and lows etc and he didn't even mention a need for a counsellor. He referred me instead to the Food Intolerance centre of excellence in the UK, which just happened to be based in Cambridge. What luck!

I went along and was given a skin prick kind of test, but, more importantly, I was asked about what I most craved and least wanted to give up. I actually saw Dr. Jonathan Brostoff personally, who was the UK expert on Food Intolerance at the time and may still be. I was put on an exclusion diet where I was allowed meat, fish, vegetables, salads and not much else for the first couple of weeks and then I had to go back and more foods were to be added in. I remember losing about 10 pounds in a fortnight, but, even more astonishing for me was that I just completely changed into a different person overnight. It was almost indescribable – but hopefully some of you know what I'm talking about, having experienced the same by ditching junk, for real food. I remember my skin being so clear and my hair shiny and everyone commenting on how well I looked. I was allowed back on fruit and whole grains quite quickly, but told to stay off dairy for some time (not sure I needed to, to be honest; I had never craved dairy of any kind).

Bingo, I thought. That's me sorted for life. I love Dr. Brostoff. However, I didn't realise at the time that there were two other pieces to the jigsaw. I replaced sugary stuff with fruit (sugar in a different form) and I got to the point that I was eating dried fruit (mostly medjool dates) by the pound, grapes by the pound, cherries by the bucket load – an obscene amount of fruit. All of this I thought was super healthy, of course, as so many people still believe today. By the time I was 25 and living and working in London, I was a complete sugar addict. The sugar had come back into my diet and I seemed powerless to overcome cravings for sweets and chocolate. Even cakes and biscuits, which I had not eaten for years, were calling out to me and I couldn't say no.

Hypoglycaemia

This was the start of probably the scariest period of my life-relationship with food. I started passing out with blood glucose lows. The worst time was on the London Underground and I came round with a kind lady looking after me on the bench on the platform, but who knows what could have happened to me or my belongings. Because of my brother being diabetic, I was continually tested for diabetes and the tests were always negative. Looking back, if I had not sorted this out within a few years, I am sure that I would have been a type 2 diabetic by the age of 30.

I went to two GP's during this time – one wanted to refer me to a counsellor again – she was extremely dismissive and unhelpful. The other one said if I felt faint I just needed to eat a Mars Bar®. Great – and then feel faint again 90 minutes later and get even fatter during the process. (I was really struggling to keep my weight under 130lb at this point – 20lb heavier than I am now at 5'2". This was only achieved with many starve days and drawing on any willpower I had left after my period of anorexia). I asked the second GP to send me for a glucose tolerance test – something I had heard about while reading as widely as I could. I passed out approximately 60 minutes into the glucose tolerance test and the daft doctor still suggested that I live on Mars Bars.

That was probably my first realisation that the medical profession do not always know best and I took my health into my own hands. I was fortunately travelling to the USA quite a bit with my work at the time and the USA turned out to be years ahead of the UK in health matters. I tended to be alone in the evenings and weekends over there so I loved wandering around shopping malls where they had coffee shops in book stores, so I would go in for an evening and drink cappuccinos and read books – bliss.

One evening I came across a self help medical section and a particular book screamed out at me: *Hypoglycaemia: The disease your doctor won't treat* by Saunders and Ross. When I flicked through the symptoms listed in the introduction my jaw was on the floor. I couldn't believe that someone had written a book that so described what I was going through. I bought the book and Carlton Frederick's *New low blood sugar and you* and devoured every word.

The clear explanations of how I had been messing up my insulin mechanism and making things worse made sense and the symptoms were all there. The solution was scary because of my sugar and fruit addiction. I actually found it easier to go cold turkey on sugar, than fruit. I had a deep held view that fruit is so healthy that I must eat it.

The recommended diet was very similar to the original Food Intolerance diet I undertook while at Cambridge, but I don't think I made that connection at the time. I tried and failed the diet many times – my addictions ran deep and there were no support groups or testimonials to encourage me. I confess that my success in staying off foods high in fake or natural sugar was not high during my mid 20s.

Candida

The final breakthrough came while reading a magazine on nutrition at the age of about 27 and seeing a nutritionist write about yeast infections. I thought that she was just talking about thrush and thought little more about it. Then, browsing through a Holland & Barrett book stand one day, another book jumped out to talk to me. It was the Leon Chaitow classic *Candida Albicans: Could yeast be your problem?* The front of the book listed "irritability, bloatedness, heartburn, tiredness, allergies, cystitis, menstrual problems" and I suddenly realised Candida wasn't just about thrush. I tracked down the nutritionist in the article and arranged a phone consultation straight away.

This Chaitow discovery was the final piece in the jigsaw for me. I took the book home and it was like a light bulb moment. In the chapters on Candida, Food Intolerance and Hypoglycaemia in this book I list all of these early works as recommended reading. They are not out of date – they were absolute trailblazers and should still be admired and read today. I treasure the originals of these books, as they literally changed my life.

I remember one weekend in my flat in London, where I lived alone at the time (being obsessed, and having problems, with food, are not conducive to having flat mates). I laid out all the books on the living room floor and remembered passages that I had skimmed over at the time. I remember reading one bit in a book on Hypoglycaemia about "your get up and go has

7

got up and gone" and bursting into tears – that had been a great description of my 20's thus far.

Time to be a mathematician – I got a pad of paper and started to write down the symptoms of each of the conditions, the causes for each of the conditions and the recommended diet for each of the conditions and the similarities were just startling.

There were passages in the books just here and there – if you didn't read the book thoroughly you might miss them. They turned out to be the inspiration behind this book. They captured in the most raw and real way what doctors were seeing when they were treating the three conditions – Candida, Food Intolerance and Hypoglycaemia. The comments on the first two of those three conditions particularly were dynamite. I share them all in the chapters on Candida and Food Intolerance and they will resonate with any food addict. The pioneering doctors, who wrote those early works on these little known ailments, had the answer to the question asked in the title of this book. From the perspective of the particular condition in which they had expertise, they would have been able to explain why their patients had insatiable food cravings, felt addicted to food and were overweight or obese. They had the answer to the million dollar question and didn't realise the potential of their work.

Pulling it all together

On more bits of paper I started to pull together the perfect diet for each of the conditions. Mathematicians will understand this as – a search for the lowest common denominator for all three conditions.

The most challenging condition was Candida, as the advice for this varied quite a bit between the experts writing at the time. I summarised where each stood on different food groups – all of the different views are summarised in the Candida chapter.

Some judgments were easy, as part of the process to try to establish 'the perfect diet' for all three conditions:

- Did they all allow real meat? Yes. Processed meat? No. So real meat is in and processed meat is out. The same outcome held for real fish vs. processed fish.

Some judgments were slightly more thought provoking:

- Did they all allow eggs? Yes, but with a caveat for Food Intolerance that, if someone has craved eggs and may think they are intolerant to them, they should leave them out. Hence eggs are allowed in Phase 1 with the note about the person needing to be honest if they have craved them.

Fruit was one of the most difficult decisions:

- Fruit was allowed freely for Food Intolerance; not allowed freely for Hypoglycaemia and not allowed for some time in the Candida diets. I decided that Phase 1, 'the perfect diet', should have no fruit, as fruit was *not* deemed OK for two of the conditions. It was clear that Candida needs to be the driver for when fruit is re-introduced. (Hypoglycaemia is also an important consideration in the fruit decision, but Candida is the most important condition).

Thus Phase 1 was born – the length of Phase 1 was determined by Food Intolerance. Food passes through us in approximately four days, so, at five days, the substances to which we are intolerant should no longer be in our systems and the cravings should be massively reduced. I tried it and they were. Bingo! This has been confirmed by so many of you since. Hypoglycaemia can be hugely helped in just one day – we can start to stabilise blood glucose levels the minute we stop eating processed carbohydrates. Candida is the one condition that is not 'fixed' within five days and people may need to stay on Phase 1 longer to really zap this horrible parasite. If I'm honest, another driver for the length of Phase 1 was that I was a huge fruit addict at the time and, personally, I couldn't bear the thought of being 'off fruit' for more than a few days. No wonder – fruit sugar was feeding my Candida beautifully.

Phase 2

Phase 2 was a similar mathematical exercise. It was partly driven by Phase 1 – what are we already eating and what might we be able to add back in to the diet for nutrients and variety. The second key driver was, having been on every diet under the sun, it was relatively easy to compile a list of criteria that the perfect diet would need to meet. The five that I thought were critical were:

1) It must work – and not just in the short term. It must help you reach your natural weight and stay there.
2) It must be practical – a real diet for the real world. No working out grams of protein or counting calories or carbohydrates – some simple rules that you can follow at home, at work or eating out, as part of your busy lifestyle.
3) It must be something you can follow for life – a real lifestyle change – something you can stick to easily and not something you go on and then go off leading to lifelong weight fluctuations.
4) It must be healthy – and deliver the nutrients you need for healthy living.
5) It must be enjoyable – and not take away eating as a pleasure in life.

This was my own check list and I invite you to do your own scoring against these criteria (you can add new criteria if you like).

Phase 2 just ticked all the things that I wanted from a diet (and I hope it does for you too). It is healthy, enjoyable, a way of life, practical and it works. The Phase 2 principles are the ones we keep for life 1) only eat real food 2) don't mix fats and carbohydrates (we'll explain why) and 3) keep those three conditions managed for you personally. That's the way to feel great, lose weight and never crave food again.

The Phase 2 rules came about from wanting to condense the principles of a lifelong way of eating into as short and simple a list as possible. The first rule was no debate – we have evolved eating real food and we have to go back to eating real food. I truly believe that every modern illness (diabetes, cancer, heart disease etc) would be massively helped, if not eradicated, by returning to eating real food, as nature provides it.

The second rule developed from connections that I made when I first started to study nutrition. The connections were between macronutrients[i], insulin and weight loss and had been at the back of my mind since my brother developed diabetes. The first observation made was that protein is in everything – with just two exceptions: oils and sucrose. Lettuce, apples, bread, pulses – as well as the obvious meat, fish, eggs and dairy products etc – all contain protein. From this it follows that, food is a combination of fat and protein or carbohydrate and protein. Since protein is in everything, we can then just abbreviate the fat/protein to fat and the carb/protein to carb.

The key distinction between the two groups is those that have an impact on insulin (carbs/protein) and those that don't (fat/protein). Back to my brother – carbs and insulin are the secret to weight and weight loss. When Adrian first developed diabetes, the only thing that changed in his body, in effect, was that he stopped producing insulin. No insulin means no ability to store fat. A type 1 diabetic will lose sugar (calories) in the urine until the condition is diagnosed, but these excreted calories cannot explain the dramatic weight loss that occurs before the diabetes is managed under medical supervision. A key observation that must be made is the massive impact that insulin has on weight. Once people start injecting insulin, they struggle to stay at a normal weight for life. Adrian has done really well in this respect, but I think it's because he's a great 'cook from scratch' chef and has always only eaten real food.

When you study nutrition, you learn how the body digests food and uses food for energy and then you realise that, the minute the body sees a carb it will use that for energy first – it's the easiest food to break down into glucose. The body is

---

[i] Macronutrients are nutrients that we need in macro (large) quantities. We know the three macronutrients as carbohydrates, fat and protein.

11

also keen to save some fuel for later on (we are evolutionarily hard wired to store food). It wants to store fat, ideally. So then you realise that, if we eat a ham sandwich, the body wants to use the bread for immediate energy and it wants to store the ham for later on. It can only store fat if insulin is present. And – insulin is present because we just ate a carb. Perfect – we have helped the body to store fat by eating carbs at the same time. Great for a caveman – not so good for a 21st century slimmer. So it just seems so obvious not to eat the two macronutrients together.

Sometimes people who have heard just a bit about The Harcombe Diet say "oh it's one of those food combining diets". Hay was the original food combining diet and this was based on the principle about how the body digests food (again carb/proteins and fat/proteins are digested quite differently). Hence Hay was more about making sure that you didn't get indigestion, bloating, bowel problems etc. It wasn't about trying to use what we know about insulin to make sure that we don't store fat. This is new and unique to The Harcombe Diet.

The final Phase 2 rule returns to the core unique aspect of The Harcombe Diet – the three conditions that cause food cravings and how to ensure that you remain free from food addiction for life. Phase 2 will teach you how to become an expert in recognising the condition(s) from which you are suffering and how to avoid the particular foods that feed those conditions. Manage the conditions and the cravings manage themselves.

Phase 3

Phase 3 has been a revelation to me. When I first started trying to work out a diet that would get me slim and keep me there for life (forgive me but I had not even thought of writing a book or sharing anything for many years after I sorted myself out), I really loved the idea that I might be able to eat biscuits, crisps, cakes, chocolates again and be able to eat them without feeling addicted.

I confess that I slipped up quite a few times moving between Phase 2 and Phase 3. I cheated too much, too often and on things that were far too processed. Hence the guidelines that are shared in Phase 3 – eat the things with the fewest processed ingredients: crisps with just potatoes and sunflower oil, not Pringles® that have 20 horrific ingredients in them. Dark chocolate with cocoa, cocoa butter, vanilla and a tiny bit of sugar – not milk chocolate, which is essentially sugar, powdered milk and other processed stuff. I also came to realise that, whereas my weight always used to determine what I ate – now the main determinant of what I eat *by a margin* is how I feel. I know that I could cheat on cheap chocolates and get away with it, but the thought makes me feel sick. I would never be that horrible to myself again.

It will only be natural to start Phase 1 dreaming of how quickly you can get back to eating the food(s) that you currently crave. I genuinely hope that, once you get to the weight and eating pattern that you desire, you no longer want any of these foods again. They are not treats – they are punishment. The realisation that I would get to the point where I despised the foods to which I was once addicted has been the biggest overall shock to me throughout this whole journey.

From helping me to helping others

The final part in the story is dedicated to Earl Lynch. Earl is an incredible motivational speaker and facilitator/trainer like no other. Earl is the reason that there was ever a first book...

I was the Human Resources (HR) Director for the Welsh Development Agency from 2002-2005 and had the most wonderful team working with me. We went on a team building session in the summer of 2003 and Earl was our trainer. We had laughter, tears and bonded in a way some of you may understand, if you have been on similar sessions with work or community clubs.

At the end of the session we buddy'd up and made a promise to our buddy about something we had always longed to do, but had never gotten round to. I was teamed up with

13

"Sian", a young HR trainee destined for HR manager and more. Sian said that she was going to get fit for the first time in her life, as she was ashamed that she got puffed out running for a bus. I said that I would love to write a book to help other people addicted to food, but I would try to think of something more achievable because I would never do that. Earl happened to be passing our seats as I said that. Like any great facilitator, he intervened. "What's stopping you?" he gently asked. "Time", I said "I would never get the time to write a book." Earl then said "I've heard you guys all talking about Big Brother – you seem to have the time to watch that..." and then he walked away.

Talk about hitting home. I thought about all the time I wasted doing things that were really of no value in my life. I then committed to Sian that I would write the book.

That August, my husband, Andy, and I went on the first two week holiday that we had had. Instead of taking the usual half a dozen 'chick lit' books, I took a lap top. I decided whenever I would normally read, I would write instead. In the totally inspirational surroundings of beaches and palm trees in St Lucia, I wrote the bulk of the original version of *Why do you overeat?* I was so motivated, I spent the autumn getting up at 5am to write for two hours before heading off to work. I finished the manuscript over the winter holidays and the book was launched at the London Book Fair in March 2004. The first copy off the press went to my buddy Sian, who, by then, was as fit as a fiddle.

I put my email address in the first edition of the first book – thinking that about 20 people would read it. Hundreds of emails later I realised that people were losing several pounds in Phase 1 and then going on to lose several more in Phase 2 and keeping this weight loss off.

One woman wrote to me: Where were you when I was stuffing my face at college? And I replied – probably doing the same thing! That's when I realised that I may not be an HR Director for much longer.

Zoë Harcombe

Part One

****

Why do you overeat?

Chapter Two

∗∗∗∗∗∗∗∗∗∗∗∗∗

Why do you overeat?

Good days and bad days

There is a current epidemic of overeating. Millions of people in the developed world are waking each morning wondering whether the day will be 'good' or 'bad'. We are not thinking about the weather, or about what we will do at work or leisure. We are thinking about what and how much we will eat.

On a 'good' day we will get through the time from when we get up to when we go to bed without overeating. The relevant words here are 'get through'. The day is never easy. Rather it is a constant battle of resistance, a continuous struggle against the urge to eat. Some people will go to great lengths to lessen the temptation – even to the extent of staying in bed or taking a trip into the countryside away from shops. I still remember a tragic story, which made headlines in the UK in the 1980s, about a bulimic aerobics teacher who faked her own disappearance one December rather than face all the overeating opportunities that Christmas gives. How many of us can empathise with her extreme measures? Any reader familiar with the 'good' day scenario will know that it ends with a sense of achievement but also an underlying fear that the period of being in control with food is likely to be short-lived. This is invariably the case.

On a 'bad' day we will *not* be able to resist the urge to eat and, having started, we may not be able to stop. Many overeaters eat so fast that they do not taste the food. Most rarely enjoy much more than the first mouthful, if that. Many eat way beyond the feeling of fullness. Many continue to eat even when they feel bloated or even physically sick. Yet we want more than anything else to be slim. Magazines ask which we would rather happen: to be and stay at our ideal weight for life; to win the lottery; to meet the partner of our dreams; or to land our dream job. Guess what comes top? How can we question the desire to be slim? It is at the top, heading the list, of the most desirable things in the world.

We are prepared to risk our lives in the pursuit of our goal. We will have our stomachs surgically altered so that the gut, called the second brain of the body, can no longer function properly. We will take tablets, the full consequences of which we know not, in the desperate hope that they will be magic pills. We will avoid food altogether and drink manufactured 'food' replacement 'shakes' for months on end, not caring if vital fat protecting our organs is lost – so long as the more visible fat disappears. We do all of this because our desire to be slim knows no bounds. And yet more of us than ever are overweight and the numbers are rising at an alarming rate. The one conclusion you have to reach is that what we are currently doing doesn't work. Counting calories, fad diets, slimming pills are clearly not the answer or obesity would not be an issue, let alone an epidemic. Why, why, why, therefore, do we overeat?

Why do you overeat? When all you want is to be slim

For too long the answer offered has been a psychological one – many overeaters are females and so the mother-daughter relationship has been seized upon by a host of post-Freudian writers. The issue of women's sexuality in the late twentieth/early twenty-first century has been discussed at length – the role of the supermodel and our magazine culture. Men are now also believed to be caught up in this magazine culture and under pressure to achieve a certain look. We are in the period of the greatest change known to humankind and the stress that this has caused has also been cited as a reason for our inability to follow a healthy eating plan. Many other suggestions have been made in an attempt to explain why, in developed societies, so-called-healthy food is more widely available than it has ever been and yet obesity and overeating are at record levels.

The psychological reasons behind overeating have a place in the theory of the condition, but they are not sufficient as explanations. There is a lot going on psychologically when we overeat but, as I will set out in this book, far more important is what is going on physically. The willpower needed by overeaters to resist the urge to binge is so intense that it cannot be less than the desire an alcoholic has for a drink or a smoker has for a cigarette. Yet overeaters are treated as people with no willpower at best or a psychological condition at worst. Why are alcoholics and smokers treated as addicts with a physical problem (and possible secondary emotional problems) when overeaters are seen as people with a psychological disorder? Why are overeaters also not seen as addicts, just like alcoholics or drug addicts?

The answer to the question that is the title of this book is that you overeat because you are a food addict. Your cravings for food, which drive you to overeat, are as strong as those cravings experienced by drink or drug addicts. At the exact moment you overeat, your desire to eat is stronger than even your immense desire to be slim. You do desperately want to be slim. You wake up determined, you stick to a diet for a couple of hours or days but then you have a craving so overwhelming that you will drive to any store that is open in the middle of the night, or you will eat the children's sweets, or you may even take things out of the dustbin that you threw away yesterday to stop you eating them. You are *not* a failure. You are not greedy or weak-willed. None of this is your fault. You are addicted to food. You can, however, change this.

What is (food) addiction?

Addiction to a substance has four main characteristics:

1) An uncontrollable craving.

2) Increasing tolerance so that more of the addictive substance is needed in order to produce the same effects.

3) Physical or psychological dependence – consumption of the substance produces a feeling of wellbeing (euphoria in the

extreme) when you first consume it and then, in the latter stages of the addiction, the substance is needed to avoid unpleasant withdrawal feelings.

4) Adverse effects on the consumer.

Food addicts will empathise with the above – let us look at the four characteristics of addiction using chocolate as an example:

1) 'Chocoholics' will describe cravings for chocolate that are addict-like and quite uncontrollable.

2) The chocolate binges get worse and worse and 'chocoholics' feel the need to consume ever-increasing quantities of chocolate to satisfy their addiction.

3) The third characteristic – physical or psychological dependence – describes the situation where the addict stops getting good feelings when they eat chocolate. They actually get to the point where they need chocolate to stop the withdrawal symptoms, i.e. they need chocolate not to feel good but to stop feeling bad.

4) Finally, think about the adverse effects – the unbearable cravings, the dopey feelings, headaches, bloating, weight gain/fluctuations, water retention, fatigue and so on. If it were not for these you would have little reason to confront the problem – you would just carry on eating chocolate. But food addiction gets worse, not better and at some stage the adverse effects get so bad that you have to act.

In the above respects food addiction is exactly the same as alcoholism or drug addiction. Drug addicts get a fantastic high when they first take, say, heroin. Then, perhaps for a few occasions while taking the substance, they experience great highs. Very quickly, more quickly with some people than others, the highs wear off and the drug is then needed not to get high but to avoid the equal and opposite low, which becomes more and more unbearable. The craving for heroin becomes insatiable and more and more of the substance is needed to continually avoid the terror of the withdrawal symptoms. The adverse effects on the consumer at this stage are dreadful – tracks on the arms, tremors, sweats, severe weight loss, no energy, no sense of life, let alone zest for life, pale skin, shattered immune system, infections and possibly even HIV if needles have been shared.

Food addiction differs from drug addiction only in the extreme lengths people will go to for their fix and perhaps in the strength of the adverse effects. In general, drug addiction leads to more physical and mental damage than food addiction. However, if you have seen a 200-300 pound person with no energy or health or desire for life, existing day to day rather than living, you may wonder that there is little difference in the effect that food or heroin can have on our wellbeing. Drug addicts will commit crime for their fix, but maybe this is only because of the price of the substance. If chocolate cost hundreds of dollars for an ounce what would addicts do to get their fix? I have heard chocolate addicts joke that they would "mug an old lady" for a confectionery bar – perhaps there is a dark undercurrent to the joke!

Food addiction is absolutely devastating – it leads to the good and bad days described earlier. It can lead to the addict thinking of nothing but food from the minute that they wake until the minute that they go to bed, with every day being a battle of wills – fighting what you want to eat with what you think you should eat. Some days you win the fight, some days you don't.

To be a food addict means to no longer have control over your food consumption. Depending on the degree of your addiction it can also mean some, or all, of the following:

- To be obsessed with, yet terrified of, food.
- To think about food from the minute you wake up until the minute you fall asleep.
- To be terrified of putting on weight.
- To fear social situations where you may not be able to determine what food may be on offer.

- To decline social invitations for this reason.
- To decline social invitations because you want to lose weight before seeing so-and-so again.
- To judge a day purely by the amount of food you have, or have not, consumed, not by what you have done or achieved.
- To be overwhelmed with guilt for eating an apple if you vowed not to eat an apple that day.
- To hate yourself.
- To feel a failure.
- To decline a dinner invitation as you don't intend to eat that day.
- To decline a dinner invitation for the above reason and then stuff yourself for the entire evening instead.
- To make a fresh start each and every day.
- To be utterly demoralised by continuous failure.
- To lose all faith and confidence in yourself.
- To feel that you are having a nightmare that will never end.
- To waste vast amounts of potential because all your energy and ambition is being channelled into eating or not eating.
- To be unable to sleep some nights due to genuine hunger.
- To collapse into a heavy sleep after a binge and to wake the next morning puffy eyed, bloated, hungover and fat.
- To have two wardrobes.
- To be unable to plan ahead because you don't know what weight you will be and hence you won't know if you will even want to attend a social occasion, let alone what you will wear.
- To continually set yourself tougher and tougher 'rules' in an attempt to control your behaviour.
- To feel totally out of control nonetheless.
- To hate the lies and deception which accompany food addiction as you try to avoid food or social occasions.
- To want to be open but to feel the world will despise you.
- To put off living until tomorrow "when I'll be slim."
- To exist not to live.

If you empathise with any, or all, of the above statements this book is for you. The above list describes a nightmare – the most horrible place to be. I wrote the above list back in the 1980s when my eating was out of control. I read the list now and struggle to empathise with it at all but I am so glad that I kept the notes I wrote then to remind me of a place I never want to return to. To be a healthy, slim person living inside a fat body is literally to feel that you cannot live with yourself. You want to escape your body and leave the fat that you loathe so much behind. The pain and despair faced by food addicts knows no limits.

But there is a way out. There is a way to stop the food addiction and to stop the overeating. This is what this book is about. So how do we overcome this? What does food addiction tell us about why we are overeating? The message for overcoming overeating is this – you will continue to overeat, that is to crave food uncontrollably, unless you identify and avoid all foods to which you are addicted. I'll repeat this again as it really is so important – *you will continue to overeat, that is to crave food uncontrollably, unless you identify and avoid all foods to which you are addicted.*

However, saying that we overeat because we are food addicts is a bit of a tautology – it is just saying the same thing in a different way. It would be like saying we are alcoholics because we crave alcohol. Or, we are drug addicts because we crave drugs. So what we really need to answer, to get to the crux of the issue is – why are we food addicts? Why do we overeat? *Why do you overeat? When all you want is to be slim.*

Why are you a food addict?

There are psychological reasons which lead people to become dependent on food. Food does act as a comfort, a stress release, an escape. Food is like alcohol to many overeaters – when we binge we are so 'spaced out' we may as well be drunk – this may be our way of coping with the world. We do need to be aware of, and deal with, any psychological factors that may be playing a part in our overeating. However, much stronger than this, there are physical reasons for overeating and Part Three of this book is devoted to these.

You overeat and binge compulsively because of one thing that you are doing and because of one, or all, of three conditions that you may have. The one thing that you are doing is calorie counting (by this I mean trying to eat fewer calories than your body needs) and this book will show how this leads directly to overeating by itself. There are then three conditions that you may have, which lead to immense food cravings, and these are Candida, Food Intolerance and Hypoglycaemia. You will also see how calorie counting contributes to Candida, Food Intolerance and Hypoglycaemia so you will see how calorie counting both directly and indirectly leads to food addiction.

You may have one, or all, of these conditions and any, or all, of them will lead to addict-like cravings. You are not weak-willed. You are not greedy. You have a health problem, or a number of health problems, and you must think of yourself as similar to a diabetic in that there are certain foods that you simply must avoid for your health. You are an alcoholic with food in place of alcohol. You are a nicotine addict with food in place of cigarettes.

Having compared food addiction to drink or drug addiction, there is a key factor which makes the treatment of an eating problem far more difficult than that of a drink or drug addiction. The problem is this – an alcoholic is advised to go 'cold turkey' (to totally avoid drink) just as a smoker has to totally avoid cigarettes. Indeed reformed alcoholics stick tightly to the principle 'one day at a time' and they think just one taste of alcohol could set them back on the downhill path to alcoholism. The problem for the food addict is that they cannot go 'cold turkey' (excuse the pun) on food. Overeaters have to eat but not binge. That is like telling a drug addict to have some heroin each day but not too much! A sure recipe for failure.

Many overeaters would agree that it is easier to ban food totally than it is to eat it in moderation. The continued success of liquid diets since the 1980s supports this – many overeaters find it easier to survive on fewer than 500 calories a day, all in liquid form, than to eat real food on a calorie counted diet.

The current advice on overeating seems to be to eat everything in moderation. Many slimming clubs tell us we can eat anything, but we have to count the points allocated to each food (another way of counting calories). With calorie counting, we are told we can eat anything so long as we don't exceed a certain number of calories a day. We are told that no food is a sin, no food is bad for us and if we ban foods we will simply crave them. Why don't we advise the alcoholic to have a glass of wine and a measure of spirits, but not a whole bottle of either? Why don't we say to the smoker don't give up cigarettes or you will only crave them? This advice would be simply crazy for drink or drug addicts so how, therefore, can it possibly work for the overeater?

The fundamental issue is that food addiction is not seen as a similar problem to any other addiction. It is widely accepted that drugs, alcohol and cigarettes are addictive, but it is less widely accepted that food can be addictive (although caffeine is being increasingly recognised as an addictive substance). However, in many ways, your problem is worse. An alcoholic can overcome their problem by avoiding alcohol altogether. A nicotine addict must give up cigarettes. A drug addict must stop taking drugs. You, a food addict, cannot stop eating. You have to learn to live with food and to eat in such a way that you don't overeat and, most importantly, that you don't have an uncontrollable desire to overeat. Fortunately, there is a way to do this…

You don't stop eating, but you do stop eating the foods that contribute to the conditions that are causing your cravings. We will see in this book how to identify the conditions from which you may be suffering and the foods that, therefore, you need to avoid. Many of the conditions are caused by having a weakened immune system and they further weaken the immune system, in a vicious circle, once they take hold. Hence, if you can break out of the vicious circle and start improving your immune system you will be able to re-introduce foods in the

24

future which are currently causing you problems. You must stop eating the foods that are making you overeat and overweight *now*, but you won't have to give them up forever.

In the chapters on Candida, Food Intolerance and Hypoglycaemia there are explicit passages from many books that refer to addict-like food cravings. These books all identify specific food cravings as cardinal signs of Candida, Food Intolerance and Hypoglycaemia. Yet such information remains exclusive to books on these conditions and is rarely found in books on eating disorders. Why? We are led to believe that eating disorders are psychological disorders and not physical disorders. However, the medical evidence for food cravings, in relation to Candida, Food Intolerance and Hypoglycaemia, seems indisputable and the overeater can benefit so much from being aware of the physical factors that may be causing their irrational behaviour.

What is the way out?

The first thing that you have to do is to stop calorie counting. Before you panic and throw this book away, ask yourself why you are reading it. Has calorie counting worked for you? Have you lost weight and kept it off? Are you at your ideal weight and are you free from food cravings? No!

Please read Chapter Three on calorie counting before you try to hang on to this 'comfort blanket' any longer. Calorie counting has got you into the mess that you're in now and stopping it is the only way out. Not only does calorie counting not work, it leads directly and indirectly to food cravings, which is the reason why you overeat. You have to stop counting calories if you want to lose weight. Have faith, dare to try something different and please keep reading. You know yourself that calorie counting doesn't lead to sustained weight loss, otherwise you wouldn't be reading this book.

The second thing that you have to do is to understand which of the three conditions you are suffering from, identify the foods that contribute to these conditions and stop eating these foods. You don't go 'cold turkey' on food but you do go 'cold turkey' on the foods that are contributing to your addict-like cravings. There are bad foods. Some food is good for you and some is not and you have to start nourishing your body, not stuffing and starving it. You also have to stop trying to be an addict in moderation. You are trying to stop being a smoker by having a few cigarettes a day. You are trying to stop being an alcoholic by having a couple of glasses a day. Eating what you crave in moderation really is that crazy. The sooner you stop trying to (quite literally) have your cake and eat it, the sooner you will free yourself from cravings and be able to control your eating.

Who is this book for?

This book is for anyone who wants to lose weight. It is especially for those who want to lose weight so desperately that they can't think what they would like more than this. It is for anyone who has ever calorie counted, lost weight, put weight back on or put more back on than they first lost. It is for anyone who has food cravings or feels that they are addicted to food in some way. It is for anyone who will go out of their way, day or night, to get the food that they are craving. In short this book is for you, if you can't understand why you overeat when all you want is to be slim.

How can this book help?

By explaining the one thing that you are doing to virtually guarantee you will overeat – trying to eat less.
By sharing with you the three key physical reasons for your overeating – Candida, Food Intolerance and Hypoglycaemia.
By helping you to identify which of these may be issues for you and how you overcome them.
By explaining how calorie counting has got you to where you are today.
By giving you the chance to eat to live rather than living to eat.
By giving you a lifelong eating plan which will help you:

- Lose weight and keep the weight off;
- Overcome cravings for good;

- Gain energy and better health;
- Stop starving and bingeing;
- Get on with your life rather than calorie counting all day long.

You are not weak-willed. It is not your fault that you are overweight or that you overeat. You are up against some physical cravings that are quite overwhelming. Take the first step to fighting them and read this book. It will help you achieve all of the above and more. More energy, better health and a life free from food addiction.

Part Two of this book will explain why calorie counting has not worked for you so far and never will. You need to *stop* eating less to lose weight and this is going against everything you have held true thus far, so we need to spend some time explaining this principle to get you on board.

This section of the book will introduce some nutritional terms in the simplest possible language. To understand how to lose weight we need to understand things like:
- What is food?
- How does the body turn food into energy?
- Or, perhaps more importantly, how does the body turn food into fat?
- Why is insulin called the fattening hormone? and more...

We will keep the jargon to the minimum but there are some medical terms that will really help you to understand why you overeat and why you are overweight.

Part Three is the unique aspect of The Harcombe Diet. As the introduction explained, the diet came about trying to answer the million dollar question that is the title of this book. Part Three will take you through the three conditions that I discovered while trying to answer this question. We will explore the conditions, which you may have heard of – Candida, Food Intolerance and Hypoglycaemia – and show how they all fit together and all explain the many health problems that you may have been experiencing.

- What is Candida? What is Food Intolerance? What is Hypoglycaemia?
- What are the links between Candida, Food Intolerance and Hypoglycaemia?
- How does overeating link in with all of them?
- What are the symptoms? How are they caused? How can they be controlled?
- What is addiction? How does it relate to Candida, Food Intolerance and Hypoglycaemia?

Part Four will present the perfect diet to overcome these three conditions and therefore to overcome food addiction, food cravings and to kiss goodbye to overeating. This is a lifestyle rather than a diet and each phase of The Harcombe Diet will give you the tool kit to eat without hunger or cravings again.

Part Five explores the psychological reasons for overeating. The essence of The Harcombe Diet is that we cannot overcome overeating until we overcome the three conditions causing insatiable food cravings. However, for many people this is not enough. Food has become a friend, an enemy, a crutch, a life support, a full time job, a fear. Food has become so many things, for so many different reasons, that we need to devote the major part of this book to understanding why we may still overeat even when we have overcome our physical addiction to food.

Part Five, therefore, looks at the psychological aspects of overeating:

- What are the six basic human emotions?
- How do these drive when you eat and/or overeat?
- What impact has childhood had on the way you view food?
- How can you overcome any damaging impact of early messages? How can you manage family situations today?
- When you are free from food addiction and can make a real choice about what you eat – what will you choose?

Quick summary of Chapter Two

- Our desire to be slim is unquestionable – there must be something even more powerful going on to stop us achieving this goal. There is. The 'more powerful thing' is food addiction.

- While psychological reasons for overeating are important to understand, there are physical reasons that are just as important, if not more so.

- We overeat because we are food addicts, with addict-like cravings.

- We have addict-like cravings because of calorie counting/not eating enough (which makes us crave any food) and because of Candida, Food Intolerance and/or Hypoglycaemia (which make us crave specific foods).

- The only way to stop overeating is to stop the cravings.

- Addiction has four distinct characteristics: 1) an uncontrollable craving; 2) a need to consume ever-increasing quantities of the substance to satisfy the addiction; 3) the occurrence of physical and/or psychological dependence and 4) adverse side effects.

- Food addiction is just like cigarette, drug or alcohol addiction. It differs, and then only marginally, in the lengths some people will go to to feed their addiction. No one would tell an alcoholic or drug addict to drink or inject in moderation. To give such advice to food addicts is equally ludicrous.

- Alcoholics and drug addicts are advised to go 'cold turkey'. You cannot stop eating food but you can stop eating the foods to which you are addicted.

- You will continue to overeat, to crave food uncontrollably, unless you identify and avoid all foods to which you are addicted.

Part Two

****

Diet & Nutrition 101

Part Two

✻✻✻✻✻✻✻✻✻

Diet & Nutrition 101

Introduction

One of the things that people most seemed to like about the original version of *Why do you overeat? When all you want is to be slim* was the nutritional information. The educated reader wants to know *why* something is being advised and the rationale behind each statement and not just to follow advice without reason. (The people who like to follow advice blindly are following government instructions to "base their meals on starchy foods" and that's why we have an obesity epidemic).

For this revised version, I have thought about what you need to know to embrace the new way of eating that is being proposed to you in this book. I think that the following will give you the foundations of knowledge, so that you can have the confidence to let go of calorie counting and eating less and so that you don't fear any of the foods that The Harcombe Diet embraces. Part Two, therefore, contains the following:

Chapter Three: Why you must stop calorie counting.

Chapter Four: What is food? How does the body use it?

Chapter Five: How do we gain or lose weight?

Chapter Three

****

Why you must stop calorie counting

In a study of formerly obese people, researchers at the University of Florida found that virtually all said that they would rather be blind, deaf or have a leg amputated than be obese again.[1] That is the extent of our desire to be slim and yet two thirds of people in the UK, USA and Australia are overweight and one quarter obese.[ii] Why?

To be slim, to achieve the thing we want more than our sight, hearing, or mobility, we are told that we just need to "eat less and/or do more." Quite specifically, the advice is "One pound of fat contains 3,500 calories, so to lose 1lb a week you need a deficit of 500 calories a day."[2]

So, why don't we just follow the advice? Why on earth do we have an obesity problem, let alone an epidemic, when we so desperately want to be slim?

I set out to answer that question in the late 1980's and my academic book, *The Obesity Epidemic: What caused it? How can we stop it?*[3] presents the findings of that quest. I'm going to share with you some of the key discoveries now.

The Calorie Theory

The public health advice in the UK and the advice from the USA National Institutes of Health is essentially to "eat less, do more." Quite specifically, the dietary advice from the British Dietetic Association (BDA) is:

"One pound of fat contains 3500 calories, so to lose 1lb a week you need a deficit of 500 calories a day."

[ii] Overweight is defined by a Body Mass Index (BMI) of over 25 and obese as a BMI of over 30.

The advice from the American Department of Health and Human Services is: (Specifically from the National Heart, Lung and Blood Institute: Obesity Education Initiative).

"A diet that is individually planned to help create a deficit of 500 to 1,000 kcal/day should be an integral part of any program aimed at achieving a weight loss of 1 to 2 pounds per week."

Where does calorie counting come from?

The definition of a calorie is "a unit of heat and energy equal to the amount of heat energy needed to raise the temperature of 1g of water by 1°C from 14.5°C to 15.5°C."

An average male needs around 2,500-3,000 calories a day for fuel and an average female around 2,000 calories a day. The calorie theory, as it has become known, says that if we eat 3,500 calories fewer than we need, we will lose 1lb. So the theory tells us to deprive ourselves of 3,500 calories for every pound we want to lose. This is where you get advice like "cut your food intake by 500 calories a day and lose a pound a week". The theory here is that seven days worth of 500 fewer calories adds up to 3,500 calories and that will be one pound lost.

The question is: where does this come from? The answer is: I don't know. (And nor does any other organisation that I asked, as you will see later on in this chapter).

The American chemist, Wilbur Olin Atwater and the German physiologist, Max Rubner developed the first calorimeter, which enabled the first estimation of calorie content for carbohydrate, fat, protein (and alcohol). In 1901, Atwater and Rubner estimated that carbohydrate, protein and fat have 4.1, 4.1 and 9.3 calories per gram respectively. (Rubner recorded the calorific value for olive oil as 9.4, so even his 9.3 was an average of four fats reviewed). Today, we typically approximate this to 4, 4 and 9 calories for a gram of carbohydrate, protein and fat respectively.

I am still trying to find the earliest reference to the 3,500 formula and then to trace it through to when it became 'folklore'. During the research for my book *The Obesity Epidemic: What caused it? How can we stop it?*, I came across a book called *Diet and Health* by Lulu Hunt Peters (1918). Hunt Peters states "Five hundred Calories equal approximately 2 ounces of fat. Two ounces per day would be about 4 pounds per month, or 48 pounds per year. Cutting out 1000 Calories per day would equal a reduction of approximately 8 pounds per month, or 96 pounds per year."

Hunt Peters may well be the 'mother' of the calorie theory. She says of the headings and text: "They are clever. *I wrote them myself.*" (Hunt Peters own emphasis in italics), so maybe she was the originator. However, no evidence was given in *Diet and Health* for the assertion that a 3,500 calorie deficit *will* lead to a one pound weight loss each and every time and I have found none elsewhere.

The theory

It all sounds so compelling and simple – if you need to lose weight you just have to eat less and do more. Every piece written on obesity and weight loss, from government publications to national newspapers will sum up how to lose weight as "eat less and/or do more" – create a calorie deficit. They rely on the formula that we will tear apart in this chapter – eat 1,000 fewer calories a day and it doesn't matter what your starting weight is, or gender, or genetics, or dieting history – you *will* lose two pounds a week, week in, week out, in a straight line indefinitely for as long as you continue to eat 1,000 fewer calories than you need. I should be able to repeat the diet of my teen years today and become weightless over the next year. It really is that absurd.

The ultimate naivety in the world of dieting is that the body cannot and does not adjust to a calorie deficit. The body can adjust and it does. It takes just days for weight loss to slow down. Within weeks, not months, we invariably plateau and we can get to the point where we gain weight eating the amount that used to lose us weight. The body's job description is to keep us alive and when faced with a life threatening attack (insufficient food because someone started a calorie reduced diet), the body will fight back.

Here are 10 reasons why you must stop calorie counting:

Reason 1 – one pound does not equal 3,500 calories

The whole notion of calorie counting is founded on claims that have no evidence base. We assume that one pound equals 3,500 calories and that we will lose one pound if we create a deficit of 3,500 calories but we have absolutely no idea where this formula came from, no evidence for the numbers and no proof for the formula.

The first part of the calorie formula is the assertion that one pound of fat contains 3,500 calories. You will struggle to find anyone who can demonstrate the precise calculation behind this, so I'll offer this as a suggestion:

1) One pound equals 454 grams (decimal places aside, this is a fact).

2) Fat has nine calories per gram (this is the universally accepted conversion, but it is an estimate and significantly rounded down from even the original estimate).

3) Human fat tissue is approximately 87% lipid (this is a widely accepted conversion, but it is also an estimate).

Putting these together, we can come up with the sum that 454 grams of body fat tissue has *approximately* the calorific energy of 395 grams of pure fat (454 grams x 87%), that is 3,555 calories (395 grams x 9).

3,555 is close enough to 3,500 you may think, until you see the absurdity of how precisely the formula is applied. According to those who believe this formula, this difference of 55 calories (in this case from the calculation being approximate) would make five to six pounds difference a year. The National Obesity Forum web site states "one less (sic) 50 calorie plain biscuit per day could help you lose 5lbs (2.3kg) in a year – and one extra biscuit means you could gain that in a year!"[4] No it won't. I can't even get an estimate of the formula to closer than 55 calories 'out'. Even if the 3,555 were correct (and it isn't), this would mean we all need a 55 calorie biscuit, no fewer, every day or we will be five pounds lighter in a year anyway. Every person who *didn't* have that biscuit every day should have lost 141 pounds over the past 25 years.

With little effort I can find evidence in obesity journals that fat has anywhere between 8.7 and 9.5 calories per gram.[5] The same (1911) obesity journal that says that human fat tissue can be 87% lipid also says that it may be 72% lipid.[6]

Taking the extremes of these, we can establish a range whereby one pound of fat could contain anywhere between 2,843 and 3,752 calories. Given that it is currently held that one pound is 3,500 calories we could (according to this formula) accidentally gain six stone (84lb) every year at the low end of the calculation and lose almost two stone (25lb) in a year if one pound is 3,752 calories[iii]. Don't worry about any of this – because the formula doesn't hold at any other level either.

Reason 2 – a calorie is not a calorie

A calorie as a unit of energy is a calorie as a unit of energy, just as an inch as a unit of length is an inch as a unit of length. However, that's as far as this statement (a tautology to be precise) should be allowed to go. A calorie is not a calorie the minute it enters the human body.

We are indebted to three scientists for the following: Eric Jequier, who works in the Institute of Physiology, University of Lausanne, Switzerland calculated the number of calories that are used up in making energy available to the body for the three different macro nutrients: carbohydrate, fat and protein.

[iii] This calculation is done as follows: If we think that one pound equals 3,500 calories and in fact one pound equals 2,843 calories, we would gain one pound consuming 657 fewer calories than we thought we could consume. Over a year, 657 'extra' calories a day, simply from the formula 'being wrong', would add up to 239,805 extra calories and this, divided by 2,843 gives 84 pounds, or six stone. If any of this were correct, we would lose weight more easily, as we would only need a deficit of 2,843 calories to lose one pound.

He found that approximately 6-8% of carbohydrate calories consumed are used up in converting that carbohydrate into energy; the number is only 2-3% for fat, but that 25-30% of protein calories are used up by the body in breaking down protein into amino acids – the component parts of protein needed by the body.[7]

This means that approximately 6-8% of the calories consumed in the form of carbohydrate are used up in digesting the carbohydrate and turning it into fuel available to be used by the body. In contrast, 25-30% of the calories consumed in the form of protein are used up in digesting the protein and turning it into fuel available to be used by the body. This also makes intuitive sense; carbohydrates are relatively easy for the body to turn into energy (indeed they start being digested, and turned into glucose, with salivary enzymes[iv], as soon as we start chewing). Protein needs to be broken down into amino acids, which is a far more complex process.

Richard Feinman and Eugene Fine, a biochemist and a nuclear physicist respectively, published a paper in 2004 building on Jequier's work.[8] They took Jequier's mid points (7% for carbohydrate, 2.5% for fat and 27.5% for protein) and worked out how many calories would be available to the body if someone consumed 2,000 calories in the proportions 55:30:15 carbohydrate:fat:protein. This is pretty much the proportions that the UK and USA governments advise us to eat. If anything, they would be happy if carbohydrate intake increased to 60% at the expense of fat.

Feinman and Fine demonstrated that 2,000 calories in the 55:30:15 proportions ends up as 1,848 calories available for energy. While writing *The Obesity Epidemic: What caused it? How can we stop it?* I accepted nothing whatsoever – not even a calculation in an academic paper. Hence I recalculated the Feinman and Fine figure and found it to be wrong. Papers include an email address for correspondence, so I tracked down

---

[iv] An enzyme is a protein (or protein based molecule) that speeds up a chemical reaction in a living organism. It acts as a catalyst.

Richard Feinman and queried the number and he said that an error had been spotted after going to print. The correct number is 1,825 – which would only have made their point even more profound (that a calorie is not a calorie the minute it enters the body).

I then repeated the calculation for a 10:30:60 high protein diet, (keeping fat the same and swapping carbs out and protein in), and the calories available to the body drop to 1,641 calories. This is incredible. This means that two people can both eat 2,000 calories a day and the high carbohydrate person is effectively getting nearly 200 calories more than the high protein person. Anyone still wonder why low-carbohydrate diets have a built in advantage?

Reason 3 – the pathways for calories are infinite

Reason number 2 shows that calories are different the minute that they enter the body. Reason number 3 is about the fact that it is even more complicated than the work done by Jequier, Feinman and Fine. Their combined work is about what happens when we eat carbohydrate vs. fat vs. protein calories – at the point they enter the body. If all calories went on to follow an identical pathway, this might be where the difference ends. However the body is way more complex than this.

Take a simple example of me eating 100 calories of pure carbohydrate. Only sucrose (table sugar) is 100% carbohydrate, so let's say I eat 100 calories of sugar. This can only provide energy – it cannot help with any of the 'jobs' that my body does on a daily basis. I may need the energy straight away. In which case, the Jequier work tells us that approximately 93 calories will be available to me for energy. But what if I don't need the energy straight away? The body will have to release insulin to get this sugar out of my blood stream – that takes energy within the body. The sugar is then turned into glycogen[v] and I may need this within the next few hours. If I do – the stored energy comes out of my glycogen reserves, which

---

[v] Glycogen is the form in which the body stores glucose.

requires more activity by the body. If I don't use this sugar within 24 hours (because, let's say, I'm an idiot calorie counter and I graze on carbs all day long, so I never need to dip into my glycogen stores) then my body turns the glycogen into fat – more activity required by the body. If I then have the sense to cut carbs for a while – my body will need to break down the fat to get the glucose stored as glycerol in body fat – more activity required by the body. The energy at each stage consumed may be tiny – it may be more significant – we have no idea. All we do know is that the claim that you will regularly see in magazines "cut 10 calories a day and you will lose one pound by the end of the year" is the daftest comment you will ever see in print.

Reason 4 – some calories have a job to do

This one is so important. Discovering this was one of my most memorable light bulb moments.

Many web sites (and the Tanita type weighing scales) have calculators estimating the Basal Metabolic Rate (BMR) calories needed for different people. They work on the basis of knowing height, weight, gender and age. The BMR calories are the fuel needed by the body just to do all the things that the body does – keeping us alive, keeping us warm, cell repair, pumping blood, fighting infection, running the reproductive system and more.

As an example, the BMR for a 160 pound female, 5'4", aged 40, is estimated to be 1,464 calories. (This is the imperial version of the formula. Our same woman has a metric BMR of 1,456 calories. This is a significant difference if you believe the 3,500 formula).

There is an equation, which has been used since 1919, to work out how much energy above the BMR is needed for different levels of activity. It is called the Harris Benedict Equation.[9] An inactive person (little or no exercise) is estimated to need their BMR plus 20%; a light activity individual (exercise one to three days per week) is estimated to need their BMR plus 37.5%; the individual doing moderate exercise (three to five days a week) is estimated to need their BMR plus 55% and very heavy exercise (twice a day, intense workouts) is estimated to need BMR plus 90% – even this level of activity does not double daily calorie requirement.

If our average woman above exercises 1-3 days per week, her overall calorie requirement is 2,013 – close to the 2,000 calories that we often hear are needed by the average woman. This means that 73% of her energy requirement is determined by basal metabolic needs. (Please always remember that whenever we talk about calories we are just talking about the body's form in which fuel is put in – just like petrol/diesel for a car – we are never implying that we should count these units of energy).

So, if you are exercising 1-3 days a week, approximately three quarters of your fuel intake needs to be going towards BMR activities. Only protein, fat, vitamins and minerals can help with your BMR list of activities. Carbohydrate is purely for energy.[vi] Hence any carbs that you eat are useless as far as the BMR list is concerned. Visualise an operations manager sitting within your body with a check list of things to do every day: pump the heart; liver – 500 jobs; kidneys – manage waste and much more; cells need to be repaired and so on. Every time fat, protein, vitamins and minerals come in – the ops manager can direct those nutrients to things on the "To Do" list. Every time carbs come in – nothing gets crossed off the list.

This is how a calorie counter can eat 1,200 calories of largely carbohydrate (fruit, cereal, muesli bars, sweets, rice cakes, Ryvita® etc) and not lose weight. We will develop this concept in the next chapter about how we gain or lose weight. We will compare two women, each consuming 2,000 calories, but in very different macronutrient compositions. The power of calories that have a job to do must not be underestimated.

[vi] To be precise, some BMR activities involve a small amount of energy, but the distinction between BMR calorie needs being met by fat and protein and energy needed above the BMR being met by carbohydrate (or fat) will be helpful to embed the principle that fat and protein calories have jobs to do.

41

Reason 5 – counting calories makes you eat the wrong things

When people count calories they are trying to eat fewer calories than their body needs in the naive and mistaken assumption that the body will just use up fat in the way that they would like it to.

During my research, I have also shown that the assumptions that carbohydrates and protein have four calories per gram and fat has nine calories per gram are wrong. The variations for fat (as we saw in reason 1) are likely very wide indeed. One of my favourite pieces of research was done by Barry Groves showing that cocoa butter – yes dark chocolate – has approximately 5.5, not 9, calories per gram[10].

However, thinking that fat has approximately nine calories per gram drives calorie counters down the path of eating more carbohydrate. They may try to eat more protein, but, as protein is in everything, they essentially have to choose between fat/protein or carb/protein. Some super idiots have worked out that you can take fat out of fat/protein foods (also known as egg white omelettes), but hopefully Darwinism will ensure that the lack of nutrition in this approach gets its just rewards!

So, we start a calorie controlled diet and we eat carbs. Remembering back to my calorie counting days, I had no thought about nutrition whatsoever (not having been taught much of any use in school, I didn't have the mindset that my life depended on fat/protein/vitamins and minerals). I ate 8-10 apples a day (approximately 500 calories), drank black coffee in place of food and ate a 100 gram box of fruit gums every day (approximately 350 calories) – that was my treat and I made them last as long as possible – drip feeding glucose all day long. I didn't lose weight a) because of reason 4 – because I was eating more energy calories than I needed and fewer BMR calories than I needed so I just got ill, not slim, and b) because the body does try to keep us alive so it would spend all day trying to get me to eat. Many days I would give in and end up eating crisps, confectionery, sweets, bread, cereal – carbs and more carbs. It was probably only the university and work dinners, which I had to attend, that gave me any nutrients whatsoever.

No calorie counter opts for a steak cooked in butter when they could have five apples, four rice cakes, a tube of fruit gums and a couple of slices of dry bread instead.

Calorie counters, therefore, are driven down the route of eating more of the very macronutrients that makes us fat – carbohydrates.

Reason 6 – three things happen directly when we count calories

We're getting into the heart of The Harcombe Diet here. There are three direct things that happen when we try to eat less energy than our body needs:

1) We get hungry.

2) Our bodies store fat and use up lean muscle.

3) Our metabolisms slow down, to conserve the limited energy that we have, and this means we need fewer calories to live on.

Let's look at each of these, for a quick and simple explanation:

1) The first thing that happens, when we try to eat less, is that we get hungry. As soon as you eat less than your body needs, your body sends out signals to try to get you to eat. Your body doesn't know that you have read a diet book. It thinks you have landed on a desert island and have been forced into a life threatening starvation situation and it tries to look after you.

You will be very familiar with the signals that your body sends out to try to get you to eat. Physical symptoms include: shaky hands; sweaty palms; feeling light headed; headaches and a rumbly tummy are some of the best examples. Mental/emotional symptoms include: irritability; inability to concentrate; indecisiveness and an unusually high preoccupation with food. It is no coincidence that, as soon as you start a calorie-controlled diet, all you can think about is food. This is your body telling you to eat.

This alone – your body making you hungry – is enough to ruin most diets. You start a new diet with such good intentions, but you are trying to fight your body from the start and your body will always win.

Hunger has been a life saving sensation for hundreds of thousands of years. We feel hunger, we feel compelled to end that nasty gnawing experience and we head off to hunt for food. Without this drive to prioritise food above all else, we would have died out long ago.

So, we start a calorie controlled diet and immediately think of nothing but food. The human was simply not designed to have more willpower to avoid food than the drive to have food. Victoria Beckham is a rare being who seems able to sustain an unnaturally low body weight by ignoring what must be constant signals from her body to eat. This is clearly not a pleasant state or 'Posh Spice' might smile more!

Not only does trying to eat less, drive us to want to eat more, so this truism is taken to the extreme. In the extreme, where people actually try to starve for periods of time to lose weight, bingeing is the inevitable consequence of this. Newton's second law of motion is: For every action there will be an equal and opposite reaction. Have you noticed how starving and bingeing go together? The more you starve the more extreme the binges get. It becomes difficult to know what causes what. You binge, so you try to starve the next day and you binge because you are so hungry from having starved the day before. It is a vicious circle, which seems so difficult to break out of. The key is to do neither – don't starve and don't binge. Easier said than done? Not if you can break the cravings that make you binge and stop the starving that makes you hungry. Please keep reading…

The opening to this part of the book said that there is one thing that you are doing, and three things from which you may be suffering, which are causing your food cravings.

These cravings lead you to overeat when all you want is to be slim. The one thing that you are doing is calorie counting. You have to stop counting calories if you want to be slim in the long term. Don't panic! You won't put on weight if you stop counting calories. You actually need to stop counting calories to lose weight in the long term. It is *what* you eat more than *how much* you eat that is making you fat.

If you remain convinced that calorie counting is the way to long term weight loss then why are you reading this book? You know that calorie counting doesn't work. You've tried it yourself, maybe you have lost weight and then regained it, maybe you have seen friends or colleagues do the same. The definition of madness is doing the same thing again and again and expecting a different result. Ask yourself what you've got to lose by trying something different.

2) The second thing that happens, when you try to eat less than you need, is that your body stores fat and uses up lean muscle. Lean muscle uses up more calories (energy) than fat does. Back to the desert island – your body is in survival mode when you try to eat less, so it needs to 'dump' the part of you that needs the most energy. This is the lean muscle – so that needs to go first. Your body hangs on to the fat a) because it uses up less energy and b) because it is going to be a valuable reserve if you are on the 'desert island' for a long time.

This is a double whammy for you a) because you want to lose fat, not nice, toned, lean muscle and b) because the more lean muscle you have, the higher your metabolism is. So, if you lose lean muscle, you reduce the number of calories that you can eat without putting on weight.

3) The third thing that happens, when you try to eat less than you need, is that your metabolism slows down. Your body does this to conserve the limited energy that is now coming in. This then means, as with (2) above, that you will need

fewer calories to live on and you will put on weight if you try to eat the number of calories that used to maintain your weight.

Reason 7 – three things happen indirectly when we count calories

When we start a calorie-controlled diet we do the following:

1) We increase the proportion of carbohydrates in our diet.

2) We reduce the variety of food eaten.

3) We weaken our immune systems.

1) As we have seen with reason 5, if you count calories you will increase the proportion of carbohydrates in your diet. Quite simply, gram for gram, carbs are always lower in calories than fat. If you know this you will avoid fat and choose carbohydrates instead – as the lower calorie option. Even if you don't know this, you may know the calorie content of certain foods and you may know that you could have half a dozen apples for the calorie equivalent of a salmon fillet. As the carbohydrate options are always lower in calories than fat options, gram for gram, calorie counters tend to increase the proportion of carbohydrates in their diet and reduce the proportion of fat.

If you don't do your own calorie counting, but you follow a diet from a magazine, or any low-fat/calorie controlled book, the diet will automatically do the calorie counting for you. On any low calorie/low-fat diet, your basic diet foods will be fruit, crisp breads, salads, cereal bars, maybe cereal like Special K$^{®}$ – all carbohydrates. Steak, oily fish, cheese, milk, olive oil and other fats will barely get a mention in any calorie-controlled diet.

So, counting calories/trying to eat less/following a low-fat diet – are all based on the calorie theory in one way or another and they all lead to an increase in the proportion of carbohydrates in your diet.

2) The second thing that we do, when we start a calorie-controlled diet, is to reduce the variety of foods eaten. We tend to go for the regular favourites that give us 'the biggest bang for the buck' (the most food for the fewest calories). We probably have a set breakfast – our calorie counted bread, or cereal, every day. We probably have a set lunch also – a shop bought calorie-counted ready meal or calorie counted sandwich or cereal bar. We may vary the evening meal a bit more, but it is still likely to have the same ingredients in it and always more carbs than fats.

3) The third thing that we do when we count calories is weaken our immune systems. This happens in the following ways:

- Simply because we are not eating as much fuel as our bodies need, we are denying our bodies much needed energy;
- On top of this we have just seen that we eat more carbohydrates and cut back on fats. Fats are essential for our wellbeing because they form the membrane (thin protection layer) that surrounds every cell in our bodies;
- We also develop nutritional deficiencies when we don't eat enough, because we don't get enough fats, calories and we eat a limited variety of foods.

Reason 8 – three conditions develop when we count calories

Reason 7 – the indirect things that happen when we count calories – lays the foundation for the three conditions at the heart of The Harcombe Diet:

1) Increasing the proportion of carbohydrates in our diet is bad for all three conditions:

   - Candida thrives on carbohydrates, while fats have no impact;
   - The most common Food Intolerances are to carbohydrates – wheat, sugar and corn. Intolerance to meat, fish or oils is almost unheard of;

- Hypoglycaemia is directly related to carbohydrates because only carbohydrates affect the blood glucose level. Pure fats don't affect the blood glucose level.

2) Reducing the variety of food eaten is again bad for all three conditions, especially when the limited foods eaten are generally carbohydrates:

  - Eating dieters' staple foods of low calorie cereal, low calorie bread, calorie counted processed meals, fruit and sweet 'treats' feeds Candida beautifully;
  - The very definition of Food Intolerance is eating the same food too much, too often. So reducing the variety of foods leads us to become intolerant to the things that we eat too much, too often;
  - With Hypoglycaemia – eating the same carbohydrates regularly continues to have bad effects on our blood glucose levels.

3) Weakening our immune systems, by not eating enough calories and by not eating enough fat, makes our bodies more likely to get all three of the conditions. A weakened immune system leads to:

  - Candida, as it creates the environment for the yeast to multiply;
  - Food Intolerance, as our bodies are more susceptible to adverse reactions to common foods;
  - Hypoglycaemia, as our general health is likely to impact our blood glucose level and stability.

In summary, counting calories will make you eat more carbohydrates (relative to fats). It will reduce the variety of foods that you eat and it will weaken your immune system. These, in turn, all lay your body wide open to Candida, Food Intolerance and Hypoglycaemia. Get these and you will crave foods (carbohydrates mainly) like an addict.

So, start counting calories and settle down to a life of uncontrollable cravings and food obsession. Stop counting calories and start losing weight!

Reason 9 – there is simply no evidence that counting calories works

In *The Obesity Epidemic: What caused it? How can we stop it?*, I devote entire chapters to looking at the evidence from obesity journals for the scientific results when people eat less and/or do more.

Francis Benedict is often credited as being the first person to do such an experiment, in 1917[11]. In this study, and every subsequent study where a calorie deficit has been created in a human, the outcome has been some weight loss, accompanied by immense hunger and tiredness – an overwhelming desire to want to *eat more* and *do less* (the opposite of what the study is trying to achieve). Weight loss has *never* matched the 3,500 formula – over even a short period of time. It has never even come close and weight regain has been observed every time.

Although Benedict's study may have been the first proof of this, the Ancel Keys' 1945 *Minnesota Starvation Experiment* is the definitive study.[12] (For the nutrition experts among you, yes this is the same Ancel Keys who did the cholesterol studies and The Seven Countries Study). Ancel Keys took 36 men and put them on a 1,500-1,600 calorie a day diet with a moderate walk scheduled each day. They lost a fraction of the weight that the 3,500 formula would have predicted. The men turned into hungry, miserable, food-obsessed shadows of their former selves. Within six months, Keys was finding it increasingly difficult to induce any further weight loss, even dropping calorie intake to around 1,000 calories a day. Some men started regaining at a calorie level that should have seen them continuing to lose weight. Within weeks of the conclusion of the experiment, the men had regained all weight loss, plus about 10%. (Does that resonate with anyone?)

Albert Stunkard and Mavis McLaren-Hume wrote a paper in *The Archives of Internal Medicine* in 1959[13]. They had reviewed all calorie deficit studies from the first half of the twentieth century and concluded: "Most obese persons will not stay in treatment for obesity. Of those who stay in treatment, most will not lose weight, and of those who do lose weight, most will regain it." Stunkard and McLaren-Hume's own statistical study showed that only 12% of obese patients lost 20 pounds, despite having much weight to lose, only one person in 100 lost 40 pounds and, two years later, only 2% of patients had maintained a 20 pound weight loss. I think that this is where the often quoted "98% of diets fail" comes from.

The Stunkard and McLaren-Hume study was effectively updated by Marion Franz and colleagues in 2007[14]. The Franz review looked at 80 weight loss studies involving over 26,000 people and plotted the results. Weight loss for the first six months was observed and then regain occurred, just as happened with the studies done by Benedict and Keys. People were lucky to be lower in weight, by any amount, after a year.

A UK obesity expert, Professor Nick Finer, presented this Franz study at the Wales National Obesity Forum conference in 2010 with the observation that dieting at least stops people from continuing to gain weight. Do you fancy trying to eat less/do more and starving and craving food for the rest of your life just to stay at your current weight? Me neither.

In June 2009, I decided to ask the British government and health authorities, who quote the calorie formula in their words and literature, where it comes from. So, I approached the British Dietetic Association (BDA), Dieticians in Obesity Management (DOM), the National Health Service (NHS), the National Institute for Clinical Excellence (NICE), the Department of Health (DoH), the National Obesity Forum (NOF) and the Association for the Study of Obesity (ASO) to ask all of these expert organisations the following query:

"I am an obesity researcher and I am trying to find out the rationale behind the statement: 'One pound of fat contains 3,500 calories, so to lose 1lb a week you need a deficit of 500 calories a day'. Please can you explain?"

The answers literally stunned me. They are fully documented in Chapter Seven of *The Obesity Epidemic: What caused it? How can we stop it?* In summary none knew from whence the formula came; none could prove that it held in even one single study; two quoted the same study as 'proof'[15].

This study involved 12 people who were given a deficit of 600 calories a day for a year. They were an average of 4.6 kilograms down at the end of the year and the losses ranged from 0.6 kilograms to 7.2 kilograms. That's an average 11 pounds loss after one year and the range of losses was between 0.8 pounds and 17.2 pounds. Watch out for that number 11 pounds – it may be significant.

If the calorie formula worked, every single one of these 12 people should have lost $600*365/3,500 = 62.57$ pounds of fat. Not an ounce (of fat) more or less. AND, there should have been *no* range of results – everyone should have lost exactly the same (that's what happens with a mathematical formula). More should have been lost on top in muscle/lean tissue and water – approximately 15% as a guide. This means that everyone should have lost 72 pounds exactly – no differences between people. Even the highest weight loss was 45 pounds lower than the fat loss alone should have been.

This is also a study of 12 people. There are 1.5 billion overweight people in the world and we can't prove a formula using 12 of them.

Weight Watchers® funded a study done by the government body the Medical Research Council (MRC), which was published in July 2010. The Sunday Times found that Weight Watchers® paid the MRC "almost £1m" to do the study.[16] The outcome was, unsurprisingly, a very nice endorsement for Weight Watchers® from a supposed-to-be independent government body.

The results were – 772 people were studied: 395 people were simply given some weight loss advice from their doctor (the GP group) and 377 were funded to attend Weight Watchers® (419 of the 772 completed their respective programme).[17] The study was a year in length and the likely deficit was at least 1,000 calories per day (a typical Weight Watchers® allowance in 2010 was 18-20 points, which approximated to 900-1,000 calories vs. an average 2,000 calorie requirement for a woman). The article reported that the GP group lost an average of six pounds and the Weight Watchers group lost an average of 11 pounds. There's that 11 pounds again.

The Weight Watchers® group should have lost 104 pounds in fat alone. This study provided irrefutable proof that the calorie theory is wrong, which should have been front page news in itself, but this was not the story of the article. The story was "you'll lose twice as much weight with Weight Watchers." The headline should more accurately have been "Weight Watchers® works better than just going to the GP, says study funded by Weight Watchers®; but you will be lucky to lose one tenth of your lowest expectation." Not as catchy, but far more honest.

Weight Watchers® have spent £15m on a 2012 New Year's Day TV advert campaign. The advance press release generating interest in the advert said at the end that "The company launched its ProPoints® weight-loss plan last year and in just 12 months its one million members in the UK have lost more than 11million pounds between them." The maths is easy – one million members losing approximately11 million pounds between them means an average 11 pounds per member – in one year.

The Franz study mentioned above also shows that all calorie deficit options, other than the liquid very low calorie diet (VLCD), record losses of between 0 and approximately eight kilograms at six months. The average is at approximately four to five kilograms – 11 pounds again. The very low calorie diets studied showed a greater loss at six months, but then a greater subsequent regain.

This brings us on to the final point about evidence for low calorie diets. First, we cannot find evidence (and seven government/obesity organisations were invited to provide any and all that they had) for more than an average 11 pound weight loss following a substantial (600-1,000) calorie deficit for a year (and how miserable would that year be). Secondly, there is no evidence that even this small loss can be sustained.

The Stunkard & Hume research says that it won't be. The Franz chart says that it won't be – all methods of calorie deficit weight loss start regain at around six months. (The reason I refer to this Franz study so often is that it is the most recent – 2007 and it is a meta-analysis – a study of many studies. It includes 80 different studies involving over 26,000 people. Hence it is highly significant in its findings). The MRC presentation of the Weight Watchers® study shows a virtual plateau in one study at four to five months and regain in the other at six to nine months[17].

Many people lose 11 pounds in the first week or two on The Harcombe Diet – showing the power of real food with managed carbohydrate intake. Tragically there is no formula when it comes to weight loss and there is no guarantee that weight loss on real food/managed carb will be any more predictable than any other method of weight loss. However, if anything can work real food/managed carb will and if anything will lead to sustained weight loss, then real food/managed carb will. The worst thing that we can do is to count calories, trigger all the circumstances presented in this chapter and start resetting our energy (calorie) need lower than it is currently. That's a recipe for being hungry, miserable, undernourished and prone to weight gain for the rest of our lives.

The key thing to remember is that all of these studies, from Benedict 1917 to Franz 2007, were based on the calorie theory – eat less and do more. We all know that this doesn't work, or we wouldn't be reading this book. If we have lost anything, by creating a calorie deficit, it has likely gone back on and also likely more. The way out of this is to stop calorie deficit diets. They don't work, never have and never will.

So, the simple and obvious answer to the question "does this calorie counting theory work?" is no. We have almost a century's worth of overwhelming evidence that it does not and no evidence whatsoever that it does. We have also been pushing this advice increasingly strongly since the 1970's and the numbers of obese and overweight people are going up, not down. Not only are they going up – they are galloping up at an astonishing rate. Could it be, therefore, that far from making the obesity epidemic better, the calorie theory and our obsession with eat less/do more is actually making it worse? This is my absolute belief. I am totally convinced that our current dietary advice is the *cause* of the obesity epidemic, far from being the cure.

Reason 10 – what a waste of a life

The final reason has to be – we have one chance at life on earth – whatever we think happens afterwards, this is the only shot we get at being human. I have followed an avid calorie counter on Twitter for nearly two years with 'car crash' fascination (she managed to gain 13.5 pounds between the 8th December and the end of December 2011, by the way). Can her grave stone say anything other than "I spent time on the cross trainer and counting calories"?!

Surely there are better things to do than counting calories? Surely anything is more fun, more productive, more philanthropic than this? The seven deadly sins aside, make counting calories the absolute last thing on earth you would ever think about doing.

Never eat less – eat better.

Quick summary of Chapter Three

- The calorie theory states that we will lose one pound of fat for each and every 3,500 calorie deficit that we create. This theory/formula is fundamentally wrong at every level:

1) One pound does not equal 3,500 calories.

2) Carbohydrate, fat and protein calories are completely different as far as the human body is concerned.

3) Once in the body, food can follow an infinite number of pathways – being used for fuel now, or later on, being stored/unstored, and so on. The idea that we can cut calories and lose weight according to a mathematical formula is absurd.

4) Approximately three quarters of our daily calorie requirement covers our Basal Metabolic Needs. The body needs fat, protein for these needs; not carbohydrates.

5) If we try to count/cut back on calories, we eat more carbohydrates. This is because carbohydrates have fewer calories than fat/proteins. Since carbohydrates are responsible for weight gain, this is the wrong thing to do.

6) Three direct things happen when we count calories: i) We get hungry; ii) Our bodies store fat and use up lean muscle; and iii) Our metabolisms slow down, to conserve the limited energy that we have, and this means we need fewer calories to live on.

7) Three indirect things happen when we count calories: i) We increase the proportion of carbohydrates in our diet; ii) We reduce the variety of food eaten; and iii) We weaken our immune systems.

8) Three conditions develop, as a result of the direct and indirect things that happen when we count calories: Candida; Food Intolerance and Hypoglycaemia.

9) Not one government body can source the calorie formula or prove it. No study between 1917 and 2007 can prove the formula. It is a complete myth.

10) Calorie counting is such a waste of precious time.

Chapter Four

****

What is food? How does the body use it?

What is food?

The Oxford English dictionary's definition of food is:

Food (noun): "Substance taken into body to maintain life and growth; nutriment." [18]

I will make a very clear distinction in this book between real food and fake food. The latter will be used interchangeably with the term processed food. It is wrong that we should need to clarify that, when we are talking about food, we mean real food. We should own the term "food" and food manufacturers should be required to call their concoctions "fake food."

The simplest way to understand real food vs. processed food is to think about the form in which nature provides food. Oranges grow on trees, cartons of orange juice don't; fish swim in the sea, fish fingers don't; potatoes come from the ground, chips don't – you'll soon get the idea.

Real food therefore includes: meat, eggs and dairy products from animals living naturally on grasslands; fish; vegetables and salads; nuts and seeds; and fruits in season. The seasonal aspect of real food is also important to consider. Even though pineapples grow on trees, and are therefore real food, they are not natural for people living in the Northern hemisphere. For British people to be eating tropical fruits at any time of year, let alone on Christmas day, is *not* natural.

Real food is that which comes in its original form – as nature provides it. Hence fruit consumed should be the whole fruit and not dried fruit or fruit juice. Fish should be fresh or tinned fish – not fish in batter or breadcrumbs. Tinned fish should have nothing added or taken away – the best tin to select is one in water or brine with the bones included. Salmon with the skin and bones is the cheapest and healthiest form of tinned salmon – the calcium, phosphorus and vitamin D are in abundance in the fish bones.

I sometimes think that we have forgotten why we eat. We eat because there are three macronutrients and several micronutrients that we need to survive and thrive.

Macronutrients

There are three "macronutrients" – carbohydrate, fat and protein. The Greek word macro means large and these are nutrients that we (allegedly) need in large quantities. Whether we need carbohydrate at all, let alone in large quantities, is a matter of debate, which I will address shortly. I will argue that our need for carbohydrate is not large, if there is a need at all, and that the critical macronutrients for the human body are protein and fat – but that the micronutrients provided by carbohydrate can be valuable and certainly enjoyable.

The first thing that you need to know about macronutrients is that most foods have more than one. There are two interesting exceptions. Oils (sunflower oil, coconut oil, olive oil etc) are 100% fat. They have no protein or carbohydrate. Sucrose – that's the 'table' sugar that some people put in tea or coffee or on cereals – is 100% carbohydrate. It has no fat or protein. Every other food contains protein with carbohydrate and/or fat. Lettuce, bread, apples, steak, milk – all of these and every food other than sucrose and oils, contains protein.

Meat and fish contain fat and protein and no carbohydrate. Eggs are almost entirely fat and protein – they have just a trace of carbohydrate. Dairy products are mostly fat and protein with approximately 5% carbohydrate, as a rule of thumb. Fruits, vegetables and grains are mostly carbohydrate. They all contain protein and some contain fat – some people find this surprising. Nature tends to put fat in most real food because it is so vital. Fat is not the bad guy that it has been made out to be – anything but.

Other unusual foods are nuts, seeds and whole milk. Most foods tend to be carb and protein (grains, fruits, vegetables) or fat and protein (meat, fish, eggs). Nuts, seeds, avocados and whole milk have carbohydrate, protein and fat all in significant quantities. They are the most complete foods (hence why milk is such a complete food for infants).

The key things to remember at this stage are:

- Everything other than table sugar and oils contains protein;
- Things that once had a face (or come from things with a face) tend to be fat/proteins – meat, fish, eggs and dairy products;
- Things that come from the ground or the trees are carbohydrate/proteins – grains, fruits, vegetables;
- Nuts, seeds, avocados and whole milk are the only foods with all three macronutrients in measureable quantities.

This distinction has real importance for the rationale of the eating plan in this book. We will come onto this in detail in Part Four, The Harcombe Diet, as we explain why fat/proteins (meat, fish, eggs and dairy) and carb/proteins (grains, fruits) should not be eaten at the same time. Nuts, seeds, avocados and whole milk – foods that have carbohydrate, fat and protein in measureable quantities – should be eaten with care. We explain why later.

There are some foods that are so low in carbohydrate, fat and protein that they can be eaten freely, at any time, with any meals or in between meals. These are generally green foods or 'rabbit food' as we sometimes call them. They include lettuce, salad leaves, cucumber, celery and green cabbage leaves as the key examples. They are essentially water so we don't have to worry about how much, or when, we eat these.

What are carbohydrates?

It is important to know which foods contain carbohydrate. Things that come from the trees and the ground always contain carbohydrate. Only meat and fish contain *no* carbohydrate. Time for a bit of science...

Carbohydrates are divided into three categories: monosaccharides; disaccharides and polysaccharides (saccharide comes from a Greek word meaning sugar).

1) Monosaccharides are also known as simple sugars and they contain one molecule (hence the pre-fix 'mono' meaning one). They include:

- Glucose (found naturally in fruit and grains);
- Fructose (found naturally in fruit);
- Galactose (found naturally in milk).

2) Disaccharides are made up of two monosaccharides i.e. two simple sugar molecules (hence the pre-fix 'di' meaning two). Examples include:

- Sucrose (one molecule of glucose and one of fructose) – what we know as table sugar;
- Lactose (one molecule of glucose and one of galactose) – what we know as milk sugar;
- Maltose (two molecules of glucose) – less familiarly known as malt sugar.

3) Polysaccharides are made up of many molecules, as the pre-fix 'poly' (meaning many) suggests. These include two digestible forms of carbohydrate:

- Glycogen – is the form in which animals (including humans) store energy – in the liver and muscles in the body. If you are a runner or cyclist, you may well be very familiar with the term glycogen – you may even have tried to eat lots of carbohydrate to 'carb-load' your energy store room with glycogen in advance of a training session or race.
- Starch – is the form in which plants store energy – as in grains, pulses, potatoes and root vegetables.

The indigestible forms of polysaccharides are collectively called fibre. Fibre contains sugars linked by bonds, which cannot be broken down by human enzymes, and are therefore effectively indigestible. There are two forms of fibre: insoluble fibre (which does not dissolve in water) and soluble fibre (which dissolves, or swells, in water).

Since fibre is not digestible, it is not considered to provide energy (calories) to the body. This was the founding concept for the F-Plan diet, by Audrey Eyton. It was considered that, if calories were 'unavailable' to the body then people would lose weight. If you believe that weight is about calories, this may seem like a bright idea. But, having read Chapter Three of this book and knowing what weight and weight loss is really about, this will more sensibly seem like a recipe for spending time in the bathroom!

What role does carbohydrate play in the human body?

In any definition of carbohydrate, the most common word seen is "energy". Carbohydrate provides readily available energy for the human body. Yet, surely in the midst of an obesity epidemic, the last thing that (overweight) humans need is easily available energy. We can make energy from fat and will do so in the absence of carbohydrate (in fact the body will *only* do so in the absence of carbohydrate).[vii]

The nutritional debate, as to whether or not humans need carbohydrate, centres on vitamin C. All other vitamins and minerals are found in animal foods (and some, like retinol, vitamin B12, vitamin D3, vitamin K2 and heme iron are found *only* in animal foods). At the risk of killing any debate with facts, the United States Department of Agriculture (USDA) database[19], to which I frequently refer for comprehensive nutritional information, lists many animal sources of vitamin C – and in good quantities. Veal thymus, for example, has 49 milligrams per 100 grams; chicken liver 28 milligrams per 100 grams of product and mollusc clams 22 milligrams. Compare these with apples, which have 4.6 milligrams of vitamin C per 100 grams. There are also substantial quantities of vitamin C in nuts, especially chestnuts. So, there are three points to make on the vitamin C debate:

[vii] We address a possible VO2max exception in Chapter Five.

1) Our ancestors lived for 1,200 generations, an estimated 30,000 years, through the ice age, with no consistent access to carbohydrate, if any at all. Ice age aside, there would be many regions of the world where carbohydrates were seasonal at best and nonexistent at worst.

There are still populations today that live solely on animal foods. Examples include: the Saami of northern Europe, living on fish and reindeer; some remote Siberians living on reindeer; Marsh Arabs living on buffalo milk, buffalo, wild boar, water fowl and fish; the African Maasai and Samburu, living on meat (goats and sheep), milk and blood from cattle; and the Inuit of Greenland and Canada living on whale, seal, polar bears and even arctic fox.

The latter is the most interesting population to note, as this was the culture studied in the 1920's by the anthropologist Vilhjalmur Stefansson. Stefansson lived with the Inuit for a decade and his study focused on the fact that the virtually zero-carbohydrate diet of the Inuit had no adverse effects on their health, nor indeed, on Stefansson's own health.[20] Stefansson (*Not by bread alone* 1946) also observed that the Inuit were able to get the necessary vitamins they needed in the winter diet, when even the limited plant matter found in summer was not available. Stefansson found that vitamin C could be obtained from raw meat (such as seal liver and whale skin). While there was considerable scepticism when Stefansson first reported these findings, they have been confirmed in recent studies.[21] It is likely that meat needs to be raw to provide vitamin C, as vitamin C is destroyed in cooking (the same applies in cooking vegetables and/or fruit, however, and this is not spelled out in the myth that is 'five-a-day').

2) Sugar, as the most processed carbohydrate of all, requires vitamins, such as B and C, and minerals for its digestion and metabolism and yet provides none in return. It follows that our need for vitamin C would be reduced if we avoided these substances and therefore, ironically, our need for carbohydrate (if there is any need for carbohydrate for

vitamin C) would be reduced if we ate less (processed) carbohydrate.

3) We can say with confidence that, even if we need a few berries to provide vitamin C in our diets, especially in the absence of food like raw whale meat, we absolutely do not need processed carbohydrates at all and we do not need even 'good' carbohydrates in anything like the quantities advised by our governments and dieticians.

In conclusion, therefore, although we have a fundamental need for fat and protein, we need very little, if any, carbohydrate. Yet this is the macronutrient that we are currently advised to consume as the major part of our diet.

What is protein?

Protein is the 'family name' for the group of molecules built from long chains of amino acids. Amino acids are chemical compounds containing carbon, hydrogen, oxygen and nitrogen, which combine together into different structures to form the various types of protein that the body needs. (You can think of protein as a necklace made up of differently shaped beads, where the beads represent amino acids).

Just a slight digression here – when we say that something is "essential" in the subject of nutrition, we mean that it is essential that we consume it. Many substances are essential for the human body to function, but the body can make some of these (e.g. cholesterol is utterly vital, but our bodies make it – so that we don't need to consume it in food). Hence we use the term "essential" to mean anything that we must get in our diet.

I find it interesting that we haven't reached agreement on the precise number of total amino acids needed by the human body, or the number considered essential. The debate on the total number of amino acids ranges from 20 to 22. In some medical literature you will see eight amino acids considered *essential* to the body (i.e. we need to consume them) and elsewhere ten. The difference in the view on essential amino acids may be explained by a core eight, which are always viewed as essential, and a further two sometimes included in this essential list and sometimes called semi-essential – amino acids that we think that the body can make in certain circumstances.

Please remember that all amino acids – however many there are – are vital for human life. 'Non-essential' doesn't mean 'not important' – it just means that they don't have to be consumed. Non-essential amino acids are just as important as essential amino acids, as without each other, new proteins that are needed by the body cannot be properly formed.

Some proteins are known as "complete proteins" because they contain all the essential amino acids (e.g. meat, fish, eggs and proteins from animal sources are complete). Protein obtained from plant sources is incomplete, i.e. lacking in one or more essential amino acid. So, while a vegan can have their protein needs met from vegetables and grains, it is more difficult for them to achieve this, as they need to combine different plant sources. (Soya, or soy as it is called in the USA, is claimed to be a complete protein, but it is deficient in some amino acids).

The final interesting point to note is that the body cannot store amino acids, so they must be continually consumed in our food. A lack of any one of them can result in serious protein deficiency diseases. (The body can store fat and carbohydrate).

What role does protein play in the body?

The word protein comes from the Greek word "prota" meaning "of primary importance". It is impossible to describe how utterly vital protein is – we would have no cells, no structure, no human body without it.

Protein has many functions and the amino acids all play different roles in these many functions. Protein's main function is to build, maintain and repair all the body's tissue, such as muscles, organs, skin and hair. Protein is vital for roles from oxygenating blood to fighting infection to digesting food. As an unusual example, which may interest women, collagen (a term well known to buyers of expensive skin care products) is a protein and this is vital for the strength, elasticity and composition of our skin (and hair).

What are fats?

Fats, commonly known as lipids, consist of a wide group of organic substances that are not soluble in water. There are two groups of fats in which we have a nutritional interest – saturated and unsaturated. Within the unsaturated category, there are two further types – monounsaturated and polyunsaturated fats.

Saturated fats are the most stable fats (this is just a factual statement about their chemical structure). They have all available carbon bonds filled with (i.e. saturated with) hydrogen. Saturated fats are solid at room temperature. Interestingly, when our glycogen (storage form of glucose) capacity is full, the liver turns the excess glucose (from carbohydrates) into fat in the liver and it turns it into saturated fat. If saturated fat is bad for us, this could be the first example of the human body trying to kill itself! Breast milk is also high in saturated fat, so did evolution also design us to kill our offspring? I have my own views on this; I'll let you develop yours.

Unsaturated fats, quite simply, have pairs of hydrogen atoms missing. Monounsaturated fats have one double bond in the form of two carbon atoms 'double-bonded' to each other and, therefore, lack two hydrogen atoms. Mono means one and hence, with monounsaturated fat, there is one double bond. Monounsaturated fats tend to be liquid at room temperature (but solid at fridge temperature) and are the next most stable fat. The best known monounsaturated fat is oleic acid, the main part of olive oil. Oleic acid is also found in the oils from almonds, pecans, cashews, peanuts and avocados.

Normally poly means many, but, in the case of polyunsaturated fat, it can mean only two. Polyunsaturated fats have two or more pairs of double bonds and, therefore, lack four or more hydrogen atoms. Polyunsaturated fats are liquid at room and fridge temperature. The two polyunsaturated fats found most frequently in our food are double unsaturated linoleic acid, with two double bonds, also called omega-6; and triple unsaturated alpha-linolenic acid, with three double bonds, also called omega-3. Omega-3 and omega-6 fats are called "Essential Fatty Acids" (EFAs) because the body cannot make them, so it is essential that they are consumed.

It is not widely known that all fats and oils, whether of vegetable or animal origin, are a combination of saturated, monounsaturated and polyunsaturated fat. Coconut oil has the highest saturated fat content of all foods at 92% saturated, 6% monounsaturated and 2% polyunsaturated. Lard is 41% saturated, 47% monounsaturated and 12% polyunsaturated. Olive oil is 14% saturated fat, 75% monounsaturated and 11% polyunsaturated. The above are 100% fats, so we can usefully compare their composition as percentages.

Remember that only oils are 100% fat – containing no protein or carbohydrate. Butter is called a fat, but it has measurable water content and a trace of protein, so 100 grams of butter has 51 grams of saturated fat, 21 grams of monounsaturated fat and 3 grams of polyunsaturated fat.[22]

It is not just oils and fats that contain all three fats – saturated, monounsaturated and polyunsaturated. Every natural food that contains fat, contains all three fats. There are no exceptions. We cannot eat saturated fat on its own – or unsaturated fat on its own – all food with fat has all three fats. This is not widely known and, the reason that it is so important is that it slays one of the big nutritional myths – that saturated fat is bad for you and unsaturated fat is good for you. The only difference (as you now know) between saturated and unsaturated fat is that saturated fat has all the hydrogen atoms where they should be and unsaturated fat has some missing. The idea that nature has put something in food that is harmful alongside something that is helpful is surely nonsense? Nature puts all three fats in all foods containing fat for good reason – because all three are vital for health.

What role does fat play in the human body?

After all the attacks on dietary fat, over the past fifty years, it is important to remind ourselves of the vital role that fat plays in the human body. Fats serve four key purposes:

1) They provide the essential fatty acids (EFAs).

2) They are the carriers of the fat soluble vitamins A, D, E and K.

3) They supply the most concentrated form of energy in our diets.

4) They help make our diets palatable. Food with little or no fat can be quite tasteless and sometimes difficult to digest.

Fats are crucial for every aspect of our wellbeing as they form the membrane (protective wall) that surrounds every cell in our bodies. Excluding water, our brains are approximately 60% fat (lipids in fact, including cholesterol).[23] Fats also play a crucial role in cushioning vital organs, as some people have tragically found out when fat (and lean tissue) has been lost suddenly on a very low calorie diet. Put simply, with the right fats and enough of them our cells are strong, without them they are weak and prone to attack.

Let us look at these four key roles in more detail.

1) They provide the essential fatty acids (EFAs).

Starting with the EFAs, good sources of the essential fats are as follows: omega-6 is provided by meat, eggs, avocados, nuts, whole grains and seeds and their oils (sunflower seeds, rapeseeds and pumpkin seeds as common examples). Omega-3 is found in meat, fish and fish oils – salmon, halibut, shark and swordfish being particularly valuable sources.

Omega-6 deficiency may cause: growth retardation; eczema-like skin conditions; behavioural disturbances; arthritis-like conditions; liver and kidney degeneration; excessive water loss through the skin accompanied by thirst;

drying up of glands; susceptibility to infections; wounds fail to heal; sterility in males; miscarriage in females; heart and circulatory problems; dry skin and hair; dry eyes and hair loss.

Omega-3 deficiency may cause: growth retardation; dry skin; behavioural disturbances, tingling sensations in arms and legs; weakness; impairment of vision and learning ability; high blood pressure; sticky platelets; tissue inflammation; mental deterioration and low metabolic rate.
Both lists present a compelling case for ensuring adequate consumption of essential fats.

2) They are the carriers of the fat soluble vitamins A, D, E and K.

Let us look at the importance of the fat soluble vitamins. The term "fat soluble vitamins" means that these vitamins come in foods that contain fat and/or they need to be eaten with foods that contain fat to be absorbed:

Vitamin A

Vitamin A has many functions within the body. It is needed for our sight, cell function, skin, bones, growth, reproduction, blood formation and to fight infection. Vitamin A is particularly important for pregnant women and growing children. Deficiency in vitamin A can lead to: sight conditions generally and night blindness particularly; growth and reproductive impairment; increased susceptibility to infections; and rough, dry, scaly skin. Retinol is the pure form of vitamin A – the form used most easily and readily by the body. This makes for a memorable connection between retinol, the retina of the eye and the role that vitamin A plays in sight.

Vitamin A is found in abundance in animal foods – meat, fish, eggs and dairy products – and vitamin A is found in the form needed by the body, retinol, in these foods. Liver is a particularly good source of vitamin A, which is why it is such a great food for pregnant women.

Vitamin D

Vitamin D is critical for the absorption of calcium and phosphorus. Vitamin D is increasingly being studied in nutritional journals and its possible role in disease prevention is being explored in relation to heart disease, cancer, diabetes, Multiple Sclerosis (MS) and a wide variety of modern illness. It is quite possible that vitamin D is the single most important vitamin for protection against chronic, life threatening, illness.

Deficiency in vitamin D can lead to tooth decay, muscular weakness and a softening of the bones (rickets), which can cause bone fractures or poor healing of fractures.

Vitamin D is found naturally in oily fish (for example herring, halibut, catfish, salmon, mackerel and sardines) and unnaturally found in fortified breakfast cereals. Never eat 'foods' that have been fortified with vitamins and/or minerals. a) it means that any natural nutrition was destroyed during food processing and b) if you don't want to obtain the nutrients from a natural source, take a vitamin/mineral tablet and save yourself the empty calories.

Vitamin E

Vitamin E is a generic term for a family of fat soluble vitamins active throughout the body. We are learning more about the different forms of vitamin E and more of them are being found to have unique functions. The key role of vitamin E is as an antioxidant.

The oxygen that we need to breathe can make molecules overly reactive and this can damage cell structure. This imbalanced situation involving oxygen is called oxidative stress. Vitamin E helps to prevent oxidative stress by working together with a group of nutrients (including vitamins B3, C and selenium) to prevent oxygen molecules from becoming too reactive. Vitamin E protects the skin (cells) in much the same way as it protects other cells.

We hear little about the possible heart protection role of vitamin E, yet it acts as an anti-blood clotting agent and it maintains healthy blood vessels. Ironically, our demonisation of fat may have denied us intake of this vital fat soluble vitamin, which would help with heart disease – not cause it.

Deficiency in vitamin E can lead to dry skin, poor muscular and circulatory function, damage to red blood cells and blood vessels and an inability of the white blood cells to resist infection.

Vitamin E is found naturally in seeds and nuts and in oils that come from these. Hence, we don't need to eat animal foods to get vitamin E, but we do need to consume fats. Sunflower seeds are one of the best sources of vitamin E and they have 51 grams of fat per 100 grams of product. Compare this with a typical pork chop, which has 4 grams of fat per 100 grams of product or sirloin steak, which has 7 grams of fat per 100 grams of product.

Vitamin K

Vitamin K has a number of important functions, such as its role in blood clotting and wound healing. Vitamin K is very important for the health of our gut and it is being destroyed with the high modern consumption of anti-biotics, leaving humans prone to imbalance in the gut flora and resulting illness. Deficiency in vitamin K complicates blood clotting and can manifest itself in nose bleeds, bleeding gums, heavy menstruation or even blood in the urine or stools. A propensity to bruise can also be a sign of vitamin K deficiency.

After reviewing the critical importance of fat from a nutritional perspective there is only one thought that we should have in our minds: How can anyone who *knows* about nutrition put low fat and healthy diet in the same sentence?

3) Fats supply the most concentrated form of energy in our diets.

The fact that fat supplies the most concentrated form of energy in our diets is used against this macronutrient in today's modern, obese environment. It is argued in our calorie obsessed world that we should avoid fat because of its calorie content. There are two ironies here:

a) Humans would not be here today without the energy supplied by fat (predominantly from animals, but also from nuts and seeds) during evolution and particularly during the ice age and in regions of the earth where vegetation was not available. At 80-90% water and containing only approximately four calories per gram, humans would simply not have been able to get enough vegetation to survive. (If any ancient berry approximated to, say, a wild strawberry in nutritional content, Neanderthals would have needed over three kilograms of berries to provide 1,000 calories).

b) The second irony is that fat cannot make us fat – only carbohydrate can do this. We will explain this fully in the next chapter on how we lose weight. As a brief explanation for now, the glycerol backbone, which joins fat particles into a triglyceride (the form in which human fat tissue is stored), is produced in the presence of glucose and insulin – the environment created following the consumption of carbohydrate.

4) Fats help make our diets palatable. Food with little or no fat can be quite tasteless and sometimes difficult to digest.

In this carbohydrate consuming/calorie avoiding world, we have lost the awareness of the palatability and unique satiety (making us feel full) of fat. 100 grams of Special-K® contains rice, wheat (whole wheat, wheat flour), sugar, wheat gluten, defatted wheat germ, dried skimmed milk, salt, barley malt flavouring, and a number of added vitamins to give the product some nutritional value, because any natural nutrition is destroyed during food processing. This brand has 76 grams of carbohydrate and 379 calories per 100 grams of product. Most people could eat 100 grams of this with relative ease. (I work with people who commonly binge on cereal). Try to eat 300 grams of "pork chop, boneless, raw lean and fat" – calculated by the USDA database as having slightly fewer calories than the cereal and no carbohydrate content. It will be substantially more filling, and therefore more difficult, to eat the meat than the cereal.

What are the other bits we need to know about?

We need to know about the 'sugar' handling parts of the body. We need to know about the level of glucose in the blood and how it changes. The term 'blood sugar' is often used when talking about blood glucose. However, I will only use the term blood glucose when talking about the level of glucose found in our blood to avoid confusion with the sugar we eat (the sugar that we put in drinks or eat in confectionery bars etc). This 'table' sugar does have an effect on our blood glucose level but we need to keep the sugar we eat separate from what happens to our blood glucose level to avoid confusion.

Let us define some terms:

Glucose is the primary fuel needed by the human body. (It is the petrol in our car in effect).

Blood Glucose Level – Our normal levels of blood glucose are around 3.5-5.5mmol/L (millimoles per litre of blood). The USA notes blood glucose levels in milligrams per decilitre, so the range with which Americans would be familiar is approximately 65 to 110mg/dL. When our blood glucose level stays above this level the impact is serious and can even be fatal.

Without knowing the medical detail of high, low and normal blood glucose levels, you will probably be familiar with the effects. When you eat any carbohydrate, you may experience a surge of energy as the glucose floods into your blood stream – literally a sugar high. Low blood glucose **(Hypoglycaemia)** is what you may have experienced, often late morning, late afternoon, or soon after a sugar high, when you feel irritable, hungry, have difficulty concentrating and may even have slightly shaky hands.

The body's blood glucose level is crucial to our wellbeing and it is also crucial to our desire to lose weight.

The **Pancreas** is an organ in the body located below and behind the stomach. Its main functions are a) to produce the hormones insulin and glucagon and b) to produce digestive enzymes to help digest (break down) the food that we eat. The pancreas is a key organ in the digestion of food and the maintenance of our blood glucose level. In a Type 1 diabetic, the pancreas doesn't work properly and this person needs to inject insulin, sometimes several times a day.

Insulin is a hormone produced by the pancreas. When we eat a carbohydrate our body converts it into glucose and so our **Blood Glucose Level** rises. As a high blood glucose level is dangerous for the human body, so the pancreas ensures that insulin is released to convert the excess glucose to **Glycogen**, to return our **Blood Glucose Level** to normal.

Glycogen is the storage form of glucose found in the liver and muscles. The liver has the capacity to store approximately 100 grams of glycogen. The muscles have the capacity to store between 250-400 grams of glycogen, depending on your muscle mass, physical condition and regular carbohydrate intake. Liver glycogen supplies energy for the entire body. Muscle glycogen only supplies energy to muscles. Each molecule of glycogen, stored within the liver and muscles, is bound to approximately four molecules of water. Hence, for each gram of glycogen stored, approximately four grams of water are also stored.

Putting all this together, we come up with the key fact: Every time you eat a carbohydrate, your body decides how much of the energy consumed is needed immediately and how much should be stored for future needs. As your **Blood Glucose Level** rises, **Insulin** is released from the **Pancreas** and this insulin converts some of the **Glucose** to **Glycogen**. If all the glycogen storage areas are full, insulin will convert the excess to fat. If the glycogen is not used within 24 hours, this is converted to fat. This is why insulin has been called the fattening hormone.

There are two other terms with which we need to be familiar:

Glucagon is another hormone produced by the pancreas. Think of glucagon as the 'equal and opposite' partner to insulin – the other main hormone released by the pancreas. These two hormones work in harmony to keep our blood glucose levels within the critical range necessary. If blood glucose levels go too high, insulin is released to turn the excess glucose into glycogen to lower the blood glucose levels. If blood glucose levels dip too low, glucagon is called upon by the body to break down body fat to release the glucose/glycerol contained in body fat to elevate blood glucose levels. We will come back to this in the next chapter on weight loss; as the role of glucagon is absolutely critical in this process.

Before we leave glucagon, it is really helpful to note a key fact about alcohol at this stage. Alcohol inhibits the operation of glucagon. Hence, when you drink alcohol, as your blood glucose level naturally falls over time, your body calls upon glucagon to break down body fat to access some glucose, but the alcohol has impaired the functioning of glucagon. Hence glucagon cannot break down body fat to elevate blood glucose levels. This has a double whammy effect on weight: a) your body can't break down body fat – so this stops you losing weight in and of itself and b) your blood glucose level stays below normal and you body perceives this as a serious threat to health so it does whatever it can to make you eat. This is why you get the munchies on drink night and this is why that kebab van only ever looks attractive when you're somewhat inebriated.

Alcohol is not to be feared as a dieter for the calories that it contains but for the fundamental impact that it has on breaking down body fat and craving food.

The final term with which we should be familiar is **Diabetes.** Diabetes literally means "sweet urine." It is a medical condition, which has been known to doctors for thousands of years. (References to this disease can be found in many ancient writings). In people who have diabetes the pancreas does not work properly. In this situation, when diabetics eat, their blood glucose level rises but the pancreas does not release the right amount of, or any, insulin to return the blood glucose level to normal. The fact that sugar is passed through the body and found in the urine is the cast iron test for the presence of diabetes.

There are two types of diabetes:

- Type I diabetes used to be called "Juvenile diabetes" as it used to only develop in children, adolescents or young adults. However, we are now seeing this type of diabetes developing in middle aged and older people. The onset of type 1 diabetes is sudden and serious. People experience a rapid and dramatic weight loss, insatiable thirst and the situation can be fatal if they are not diagnosed and treated very quickly.

- Type 2 diabetes used to be called "Maturity onset diabetes" because it used to be developed later on in life. However, we are now seeing type 2 diabetes develop in young adults and even children. Type 2 diabetes is by far the more common – 90-95% of diabetics have type 2.

A useful way to think of the two different types is – with type 1 diabetes, it is as if the pancreas doesn't work at all. The type 1 diabetic consumes carbohydrate, blood glucose levels rise, but the pancreas doesn't release insulin to remove the glucose from the blood stream. This is why type 1 is the most serious form of the condition and people with this type of diabetes must inject/ingest insulin in some way to compensate for the lack of insulin produced by the body.

With type 2 diabetics, the body still produces insulin, but the cells of the body have become resistant to insulin and so the glucose is not removed from the blood stream as effectively as it should be. Some type 2 diabetics sensibly try to manage their condition with a very low-carbohydrate diet (it seems so obvious – if the body can't handle glucose then cut right back on carbohydrates – the things that break down into glucose). Other type 2 diabetics take medication to try to mitigate the insulin resistance and to improve the remaining functioning of the pancreas as best as possible.

I view type 2 diabetes as the body saying "enough's enough". I have had too many carbohydrates, too often, to cope with and I can't respond any more to try to remove the glucose from the blood stream that you keep chucking in. The fact that we are seeing this in children is a clear condemnation of our public health dietary advice telling us to base our meals on starchy foods – the very things that break down into glucose and require removal by the body's super sensitive mechanism.

The causes of both types of diabetes are not known exactly, but risk factors (things that increase your chance of getting diabetes) include: having a family history of diabetes; being obese or overweight; physical inactivity; older age and race/ethnicity. People with a family history of diabetes are more likely to develop the condition themselves. Overweight people are more likely than normal weight people to become diabetic. People who are inactive are more at risk. The risk increases the older you get so older people are more likely to get Type II diabetes. Finally, African Americans and Hispanic/Latino Americans are twice as likely to get diabetes as Caucasians although we don't know exactly why.

The International Diabetes Federation (IDF) states that there were 194 million people with diabetes worldwide in 2003. They estimate that there will be 333 million by 2025. The USA has 15.3 million diabetics, which is over 6% of the USA population. Only India and China have higher numbers of diabetics and this is due to the size of their populations. They have 32.7 million and 22.6 million respectively. Diabetes is the third leading cause of death in the USA after heart disease and cancer. It is the leading cause of blindness and sight defects in developed countries and is the leading cause of amputations where an accident has not happened.

5.7% of the European population has diabetes, 32 million adults. Of these 1.6 million have type 1 diabetes and the other 30.4 million have type 2.[24]

What happens when we eat?

When you eat something, your body absorbs certain substances from your food, mostly across the surface of your small intestine. As this happens, food is literally entering your body for use.

From the carbohydrates you eat, your body will absorb simple sugars, all of which either are, or quickly and easily become, glucose. From fat the body absorbs fatty acids and from protein it absorbs amino acids, the building blocks of protein. Although we can make energy from all three types of food – carbohydrate, fat and protein – carbohydrates are the easiest foods from which to get fuel. Our bodies need the simplest form of carbohydrate as fuel – glucose – and, therefore, the body turns carbohydrates into glucose as the first step to giving us fuel.

When we eat carbohydrates our body decides how much of the energy taken in is needed immediately and how much should be stored for future requirements. As our blood glucose level rises, insulin is released from the pancreas and this insulin converts some of the glucose to glycogen, a starch stored in the muscles and the liver available for energy use. Glycogen is our energy store room, if you remember from the definitions above. The next bit bears repeating, as it is so important to remember: *If all the glycogen storage areas are full, insulin will convert the excess to fat. If the glycogen is not used within 24 hours, this is converted to fat. This is why insulin has been called the fattening hormone.*

Why do we need to know all this?

We need to know these basics because the hormone insulin is of real importance in our overeating and desire to lose weight. Insulin is the fattening hormone and the amount of insulin released into the body has a huge impact on our weight levels. Think about the following:

- Do you know anyone who has suddenly developed type I diabetes? When people first develop type 1 diabetes, their pancreas suddenly stops working and no insulin is produced. It is quite common for juvenile diabetics to lose 10 pounds or more in days as the production of insulin literally stops overnight. What does that tell us about insulin and weight loss?

- Then, when diabetics start injecting insulin on a daily basis, many struggle with their weight and many diabetics remain overweight for a lifetime. Again, what does that tell us about insulin and weight loss?
- High fat/protein, zero carbohydrate diets have a dramatic impact on weight loss. This is because a diet with no carbohydrates in effect stops the production of insulin. If you eat nothing but fat and protein, for even a short period of time, despite the fact that your calorie intake may be high, you will see rapid weight loss. (I am not recommending this as a long term diet, but it does tell us how to harness this information for use in a more balanced weight loss approach).

Just think about these facts again – your body stops producing insulin and you lose weight more dramatically than with any other illness. You start taking insulin in injections and your weight goes back up. You stop insulin production by not eating carbohydrates and your weight falls. These facts alone demonstrate that insulin is an incredibly powerful hormone and an important issue in weight loss.

We don't know everything that we need to know about insulin, but we do know that it acts to control the level of glucose in the body. We also know that it facilitates the storage of fat. *As only carbohydrates trigger the release of insulin, the secret to weight loss lies with carbohydrates.* If you restrict carbohydrate intake, you reduce the production of insulin, which is the hormone that facilitates the storage of fat.

If you Google any of the above terms – insulin, pancreas, glucose, glycogen, diabetes – you will be stunned by the complexity of the workings of just this part of the human body, let alone the whole thing. You may have two reactions:

1) Complete awe at the marvel that is a human being.

2) Complete horror at what we do to these incredibly sophisticated and sensitive mechanisms in our bodies on a daily, if not hourly, basis.

The human body is a true wonder of the world. We have over 200 bones and all the muscles and ligaments needed to move this complex structure with suppleness, stamina and strength. Some of us can run 100 metres in fewer than 10 seconds. Others can walk across the globe in months. Our heart is one of the most reliable pumps on earth. It will beat approximately 70 times a minute, 60 minutes an hour, 24 hours a day, 365 days a year for over 70 years. How awesome is that? Our bodies repair themselves and fight infection. They digest food efficiently and manage their own waste production. We can fly to the moon, cause, or prevent, other species becoming extinct, laugh, cry or tap dance. We are truly remarkable. Perhaps the most remarkable feature of the human being, however, is that we can do all of this despite the 'junk' that many of us put into our bodies. In this magnificent human body there is a mechanism which is trying to maintain a blood glucose level of approximately 65 to 110mg per 100cc of blood. How the body does this at all, let alone given what we eat, is just amazing.

What is the relevance of all this in this book?

This book can be viewed as a jigsaw puzzle. You have probably heard about some, or all, of the key pieces in the jigsaw – calorie counting, Candida, Food Intolerance, Hypoglycaemia, insulin, sugar, fat etc. – this book will piece all of them together and show you that there is one consistent explanation for everything you have read. You may have read one book and thought one thing and then read another and thought you needed to try something different. You have probably read so many diet books you don't know what to believe and which way to turn. This book makes sense of the others and pieces together the jigsaw for you to make the one compelling message – the way forward to the new slim you.

Quick summary of Chapter Four

- There are three macronutrients: carbohydrate, fat and protein.

- The only foods that don't contain protein are oils (pure fat) and sucrose (pure carbohydrate).

- Remember fat/proteins come from things with faces: meat; fish; eggs and dairy products.

- Carb/proteins come from the ground and the trees: grains and fruits, for example.

- Carbohydrates break down into sugars for energy. Fat breaks down into fatty acids, which can repair cells and/or provide energy. Protein breaks down into amino acids for cell repair and growth.

- Although we can make energy from carbohydrate, fat or protein, carbohydrates are the easiest foods from which to get fuel. When we eat carbohydrates our body decides how much of the energy is needed immediately and how much should be stored for future requirements.

- If our energy storage area (glycogen) is full, insulin will convert the excess to fatty tissue. This is why insulin is called the fattening hormone.

- If you become diabetic and your body stops producing insulin, or if you stop insulin production with a zero carbohydrate diet, you lose weight dramatically. If a diabetic injects insulin or if you stimulate insulin production with a high carbohydrate diet your weight goes back up. Insulin is an incredibly powerful hormone and has a key role to play in weight control.

- As only carbohydrates trigger the release of insulin, the secret to weight loss lies with carbohydrates.

Chapter Five

****

How do we gain or lose weight?

In this final chapter in the 'what do you need to know to start losing weight' section of the book, we put together things from Chapter Three and Chapter Four to cement your new way of thinking.

It is vital that you let go of calorie counting/trying to eat less if you are going to have success in overcoming overeating and losing weight. Each and every time you waiver, and think that eating less/doing more will work, go back to Chapter Three and remind yourself that the calorie theory is fundamentally wrong at every level. Remind yourself how it directly and indirectly lays the foundations for three conditions, which are going to feed your food addiction.

Chapter Four has hopefully inspired you that the only way to eat is the real food way. You now know that fat is utterly life vital, not something to be feared and demonised. Carbohydrates on the other hand, the macronutrient recommended by our governments, is the substance that you should be concerned about. This is the macronutrient that stimulates insulin, the fattening hormone. This is the macronutrient that we should eat far less of.

Let's build on these learnings with a bit more science. Here is what you need to know about body fat and fatty acids before we have the final piece in the jigsaw to know how we gain or lose weight:

1) There are two forms of fat in the human body: fatty acids and triglycerides.

2) Fatty acids are the form in which fat is burned for fuel by the body.

3) Triglycerides are the form in which fat is stored by the body as human fat tissue (also called adipose tissue).

4) A triglyceride is three (tri means three) fatty acids bonded together by glycerol (glycerol is a sugar, essentially).

5) Fat enters and exits fat cells as fatty acids, because triglycerides are too big to move across the cell membrane.

6) Fatty acids go into and out of the fat cells continually, 'cycling' across the cell membrane. If three fatty acids are bonded by glycerol to form a triglyceride, they can't get back out of the fat cell until the triglyceride is broken back down into glycerol and fatty acids.

Keep referring back to these headlines if need be. This may all seem a bit technical on first reading, but you'll be sharing these insights with friends before you know it.

How is fat stored?

This is another way of saying – how do we gain weight? Fat is stored when triglyceride is formed, locking three fatty acids together in a fat cell. Triglyceride can be formed when glycerol is available and glycerol is available when glucose is available.

So, when we eat carbohydrates, the body breaks these down into glucose and this enables the formation of glycerol, which can lock three fatty acids together in a fat cell. The more glycerol available, the more fat can be stored. There is one final thing needed to make all of this happen – the glucose needs to be transported to the fat cells and that's what insulin does. So, eat carbohydrates and you have the glycerol ready to make fat and you have the insulin stimulated to make sure that fat can be stored. Carbohydrates have a unique ability to facilitate fat storage – otherwise known as weight gain.

How is fat unstored?

This is another way of saying – how do we lose weight? Fat is unstored, weight is lost, when we break down triglyceride and release the glycerol and three fatty acids back into the blood stream. For this to happen the body essentially needs to be in a state of low blood glucose.

If blood glucose levels drop below the normal range, the body will then look for stored glucose – also known as glycogen – to use next. Remember from the previous chapter that the body can store approximately 100 grams of glycogen in the liver and 250-400 grams in the muscles. At approximately 4 calories per gram for carbohydrate, that's 1,400 to 2,000 calories likely available as glycogen if you are a regular carb eater. That's a lot of stored fuel that needs to be used up before the body has any need to break down body fat. Can you see how the more carbohydrate you eat, the less likely it is that you need to burn body fat?

The perfect environment for fat storing (gaining weight) is to eat little and often/graze on carbs all day long. Incredibly this is the advice that we get from public health dietary advisors. The perfect environment in which the body can unstore/burn fat is therefore the opposite – eat carbs rarely, if at all. However, just because the body *can* burn fat doesn't mean that it *will*.

If you have glucose or glycogen available in the body, you will not burn fat. The body will always use carbs for fuel if they are available (glucose is a simple carb and glycogen is a polysaccharide – just a more complex carb). If you follow the current "base your meals on starchy foods" advice, you will likely have carbs available most of the time that you are awake.

This is why The Harcombe Diet has you 'running' on little carbohydrate and when we have carbohydrates – we have them as the staple of the meal – so that the body has to use them for energy and has no fat to store for later on – let alone carbohydrate left to store for later on (unused carbs can be turned into glycogen and then stored if not needed within 24 hours). Those who have tried to do aerobics classes, and similar 'non-caveman like' exercise, on The Harcombe Diet have also discovered that glycogen stores are low. This puts you in a good fat burning mode most of the time.

The Harcombe Diet way is about trying to have your cake and eat it. We still have carbs for the enjoyment, variety and practicality that they bring to our diet, but we eat them in a cleverly managed way to keep the body in fat burning mode as much as possible. We don't snack/graze (if we need something between meals, we go as low carb as possible). We eat as few carb meals as works for each of us and we develop a way of eating that is a way of life. This is not a zero carb plan to go on and then to go off (and then risk weight regain). It's a way of maximising the time you are in fat burning mode (and not in fat storing mode), without any more pain/deprivation than is necessary.

The exercise exception

Some excellent studies have been done on people exercising to see if there are other circumstances during which the body will break down triglyceride – i.e. body fat. There is a term called VO2max, which is our body's maximum aerobic/oxygen capacity. Low exercise intensity, for example walking at a normal pace, would have someone operating at approximately 25% of their VO2max. Moderate exercise intensity is considered to be "the greatest running pace that can be sustained for two to four hours" – ouch! This is often referred to as 65% VO2max. High VO2max describes the situation where a person is operating at 85% of their maximum aerobic capacity. This would involve them running at the greatest pace that could be sustained for 30-60 minutes. Ouch again!

The interesting points for us to note are that, as exercise intensity increases from low (25% VO2max) to moderate (65% VO2max) to high (85% VO2max), using free fatty acids for fuel declines. However, total fat burning increases when intensity increases from 25% to 65% VO2max, as intramuscular triglycerides are used for fuel. Intramuscular triglycerides are, as the name suggests, fat stored between muscular areas in the body. These can provide a substantial contribution to fuel needs when moderate exercise is undertaken.

However, the same researchers have also shown that carbohydrates and insulin still get in the way of the body burning body fat, even if the optimal fat burning intensity of exercise is undertaken (65% VO2max). Fat burning during exercise is impacted by carbohydrates available to the body. Montain and colleagues showed that the amount of carbohydrate eaten, how long before exercise this was eaten and the duration of the exercise are all important when seeing if exercise can even help to burn body fat.[25] For at least four hours after eating approximately 140 grams of carbohydrate, the body burns the carbohydrate for fuel rather than needing to break down body fat. Someone would need to run for 50 minutes before starting to break down body fat, if carbohydrate has been eaten in the past few hours. After 100 minutes of running, fat burning can resume, as if the exercise had not had the carbohydrates before exercise. This reinforces the fact that the body will use carbohydrates/glucose for fuel before fatty acids or body fat any time it has the option.

Unless you are planning to run at the maximum pace that you could sustain for two to four hours, for 100 minutes, you had better manage your carbohydrate intake carefully to maximise your chance of burning body fat. For our average dieter, therefore, we don't have to worry about VO2max. We should proceed on the basis that – if there is glucose available in the blood stream, the body will use this for energy and not need to break down fat for as long as this is available.

A tale of two women

Let us now put together the facts that we have presented in Part Two of this book and give you a very memorable example of why a calorie is not a calorie and why you must stop thinking that eating fewer calories will ever help you to lose weight...

Let us take two women. I'm going to call them Ms. Mother Nature and Ms Government Plate. Ms. Mother Nature knows everything that there is to know about losing weight – a calorie is not a calorie, we must eat real and not processed food and more. Ms. Government Plate follows the standard government advice – whether in the UK, USA, Australia or New Zealand. She follows the advice to "base her meals on starchy foods".

The UK eatwell plate[26], as it is called (I call it the eatbadly plate) advises people to have one third of their volume intake in the form of starchy foods (carbohydrates); one third in the form of fruit and vegetables (more carbohydrates); 15% in the form of milk and dairy products (these have a carb content); 12% non-dairy protein (these can come in the form of beans and pulses – more carbohydrates) and there is an 8% junk segment.

I did a comprehensive analysis of this plate in *The Obesity Epidemic? What caused it? How can we stop it?* and found that these volumes became quite different when compared by calorie intake. You could do this as a 'back of the envelope' estimate. I did it accurately by measuring calorie values of different food compositions. Starchy foods have approximately 400 calories per 100 grams; fruit and vegetables have approximately 50 calories per 100 grams; dairy products and non-dairy protein have approximately 200 calories per 100 grams and the junk segment has approximately 600 calories per 100 grams. This plate therefore ends up directing people to have 50% of their calorie intake in the form of starchy foods; 21% in the form of junk and just 6% of energy intake in the form of fruit and vegetables – the law of unintended consequences.

Notwithstanding this complication of the difference between recommended volume intakes and what this becomes in calorie/energy intake – Ms. Government Plate is advised overall to consume her food intake in the proportions: 55% carbohydrate, 30% fat and 15% protein.

In the following table, I have allocated Ms. Mother Nature her food intake in the proportions: 10% carbohydrate; 30% fat and 60% protein. Please note that I wouldn't actually recommend these proportions – this is just to illustrate the difference in diets based on fat/protein rather than carbohydrate/protein. My advice would be to just eat real food, don't fear fat, manage carbohydrate and the actual proportions of fat and protein will be what they will be. They will reflect what Mother Nature puts in food naturally.

	Ms Mother Nature	Ms Government Plate
Calories consumed	2,000	2,000
Ratio of Carb Fat Protein calories	10/30/60	55/30/15
Calories available to the body	1,641 (186/585/870)	1,826 (1,023/585/218)
Assume 1,500 calories are needed for BMR	1,455 fat/protein	803 fat/protein
Assume 500 calories are needed above the BMR for energy	186 carb cals (rest from body fat)	1,023 carb cals (523 stored as body fat)
Outcome	Slim & Healthy	Fat & Sick

In the table above, our two women both eat 2,000 calories.

The points to be made are:

1) If we remember back to the work done by Jequier, Fine and Feinman from Chapter Three, we know that approximately 7% of carbohydrate calories are used up in turning carbohydrates into energy; approximately 2.5% of fat calories are used in conversion and as many as 27.5% of protein calories are used up in metabolising protein. From the same 2,000 starting calories, Ms Government Plate can have 1,826 calories available to the body and Ms Mother Nature can end up with 1,641 available to the body.

2) If we remember that the Basal Metabolic Rate accounts for approximately three quarters of our daily need (and this is if our average woman exercises moderately one to three times a week), then we can estimate that each woman needs approximately 1,500 calories for her BMR. The BMR activities require fat, protein, vitamins and minerals.

Ms. Mother Nature doesn't quite have enough fat and protein calories (585 + 870 = 1,455) to do her BMR work. Ms. Government Plate has consumed barely half of the fat and protein calories that she needs. Hence Ms Government Plate could have consumed another 700 fat/protein calories and the body had a use/need for them straight away – a missed opportunity and the fast track to disease.

3) Both women needed approximately 500 calories for energy. Remember that energy can come from carbohydrate or fat. Fat is the most versatile macronutrient. Ms. Mother Nature didn't consume enough carbohydrate calories to fuel her energy needs. Her body will have to break down triglyceride i.e. burn body fat, to meet her requirements. This is exactly what a slimmer wants to happen.

Ms Government Plate, on the other hand, has twice as many energy calories as she needs, so she stores fat rather than burns fat.

Ms Mother Nature gets slim and healthy; the people eating the way the government advises get fat and sick. This is why we have seen an epidemic of both obesity and ill health since our change in dietary advice.

The final point to note is – don't ever get tempted to eat less overall even when you see this table. Cut carbohydrates by all means, but if you try to eat less, the body can and does just reduce the things it was going to do otherwise. If you eat less, the body can just cut back on Basal Metabolic Activities. It can turn off the heating system, cut back on cell repair and fighting infection etc. The body can stop the reproductive system if things get really serious (as happens surprisingly early on with anorexics).

If you try to do more – the body can again rob from BMR calories – things it was going to do that day and the body can also rob from other energy calories. You may not end up going to the gym *and* needing 500 energy calories for the day. You may go to the gym and then crash on the sofa and just do less other activity. The body can and does rob from the BMR and energy calories if you try to eat less and/or do more. The human body is way too smart just to give up fat even if it were biochemically able to do so (i.e. having no glucose available for energy).

Quick summary of Chapter Five

- There are two forms of fat in the human body: fatty acids and triglycerides.

- Fatty acids are the form in which fat is burned for fuel by the body.

- Triglycerides are the form in which fat is stored by the body as human fat tissue (also called adipose tissue).

- A triglyceride is three (tri means three) fatty acids bonded together by glycerol (glycerol is a sugar, essentially).

- Fat enters and exits fat cells as fatty acids, because triglycerides are too big to move across the cell membrane.

- Fatty acids go into and out of the fat cells continually, 'cycling' across the cell membrane. If three fatty acids are bonded by glycerol to form a triglyceride, they can't get back out of the fat cell until the triglyceride is broken back down into glycerol and fatty acids.

- Fat is formed i.e. we gain weight, when glycerol is available. Glycerol is available when glucose is available. Glucose is available when we eat carbohydrate. Carbohydrates and not calories are behind weight gain.

- Fat is broken down i.e. we lose weight, when glucose is *not* available and the body needs to break down triglyceride to release the glycerol contained within.

- Two people can eat the same number of calories in different macronutrient proportions and the metabolic advantage of fat/protein over carbohydrate/protein is significant.

- Approximately three quarters of the daily calorie requirement needs to come in the form of fat/protein and the remaining quarter can come in the form of fat or carbohydrate (for fuel). If we don't eat enough fat/protein we don't meet our BMR requirements and this can impact our health. If we eat too much carbohydrate we store any needed above energy requirements and this can impact our weight.

- The person following the government carbohydrate intake advice will get fat and sick. The sensible person eating real food, plenty of meat, fish, eggs and dairy products and managing carbohydrate intake will get slim and healthy.

Part Three

****

The three conditions that cause overeating

Chapter Six

****

Candida

What is Candida?

Candida Albicans is a yeast that exists in all of us which is normally controlled by our immune system and by other bacterial flora present in our body. It usually resides in the digestive tract and is observed in females in the vagina, or in any sufferer on the skin (athlete's foot or dandruff, for example, are generally signs of fungal or yeast infections). Candida serves no useful purpose in the body (unlike other bacterial flora such as lactobacillus acidophilus) and can, therefore, be viewed as a parasite. In many people this yeast causes no harm and lives within them peacefully. The problem starts when Candida gets out of control and does make its presence known.

Yeast exists just about everywhere on earth, living off other living things. In the right environment, yeast is capable of explosive reproduction and growth, as anyone who has ever made bread, wine or beer will know. Science has shown that a single yeast cell, given the right reproductive environment, can multiply to over one hundred yeast cells within twenty-four hours. In the human body, therefore, given the right environment, this normally harmless yeast can multiply to frightening levels and cause significant impact on our health and wellbeing.

What causes Candida overgrowth?

Or put another way – if yeast can multiply to frightening levels given the right environment – what makes our body the right environment for Candida to multiply?

There are five key causes:

1) A weakened immune system.

2) Over-consumption of processed carbohydrates.

3) Medication – steroids, antibiotics, birth control pills, hormones.

4) Diabetes.

5) Nutritional deficiency.

1) If you have a weakened immune system you are more susceptible to Candida overgrowth and in fact Candida overgrowth is often seen as evidence of a weakened immune system. One will make the other worse in a vicious circle. If you have had a period of illness, or significant personal or work stress, the chances are that your immune system will be weaker than normal and this provides an ideal opportunity for Candida to multiply. This will then further weaken your immune system.

2) Anyone who has made beer at home will know the effect of combining yeast and sugar. The effect on Candida is much the same. The yeast thrives on all processed carbohydrates, concentrated fruit sugar, yeast and yeast derivatives and vinegary/pickled foods. The fact that Candida emerged as a significant health issue in the twentieth century is not surprising given the recent increase in processed food consumption. As we have increased our consumption of processed foods, we have fed the parasite Candida in our body and enabled it to get out of balance.

3) There are many modern medicines that upset our natural body harmony and encourage the overgrowth of Candida. These include steroids, antibiotics, birth control pills and hormones, all of which were unknown before the twentieth century. This is a further reason why Candida, and the related obesity problems, have become far more prevalent in recent years. Antibiotics are chemical substances capable of destroying or inhibiting the growth of living things such as germs but they are also capable of killing lactobacilli,

which are found in the intestines. Lactobacilli are part of the 'friendly' gut bacteria which control Candida and thus antibiotics can contribute to a proliferation of Candida as the gut flora balance is disturbed.

4) As we know from Chapter Four, diabetes is also known as "*sweet urine*" and it occurs where the pancreas does not release insulin to regulate the glucose level in the blood. Diabetics, who literally have an excess of glucose in their blood, are providing the ideal breeding ground for Candida. It is well known that diabetics struggle more with their weight than the average non-diabetic and there could be a few reasons for this:

- The injections of insulin lead directly to weight problems as insulin is the fattening hormone (remember what we don't use up is stored as fatty tissue).
- Diabetics are more prone to Candida with their sugary body environment and, therefore, the cravings linked to Candida are likely to be making them fat.
- Diabetics no longer have a natural mechanism to regulate their blood glucose level and are, therefore, trying to avoid a state of Hypoglycaemia at all times by balancing injections with food consumed. They are, therefore, susceptible to food cravings if this balance is out of sync at any time.

5) There is much evidence to suggest that our nutritional deficiency has actually got worse and not better as we have 'developed' as nations. Analysis in the UK reveals that the war time diet, when food was rationed, was actually better for us than our current diet where we can freely choose from every food available. In war time we were limited to fixed amounts of meat, fish, vegetables, fruits, dairy products and grains but we were also limited in our access to sugar and other processed carbohydrates. In comparison with current diets, high in processed foods, our predecessors ate quite well. We may be overeating as developed nations but we are certainly not over consuming nutrients. A

number of nutrients are key to the control of Candida and there is evidence that they are lacking in our current diets:

- Biotin, one of the B vitamins, can help prevent the conversion of the yeast form of Candida to its fungal form. One of the richest sources of biotin is pigs' kidneys while reasonable sources are eggs and whole grains.
- Vitamin C affects general immunity which impacts the environment in which yeast can multiply. Stress also depletes vitamin C and we may not be getting the levels of vitamin C we need for optimal health and immunity with our current 'fast food' diets. Vitamin C is not stored by the body so we need a constant supply to keep Candida at bay.
- B vitamins are also needed for stress tolerance and the immune system and we lose valuable sources of B vitamins when we opt for processed carbohydrates over real food, especially meat, fish, eggs and dairy products. Cereals and breads are often fortified with added vitamins and these are the only sources of B vitamins in many of our diets. However, these come in products laden with sugar and other processed carbohydrates so we would be better off avoiding them altogether and eating real foods rich in natural nutrients, or taking a vitamin pill on its own.
- Magnesium, selenium and zinc are the key minerals needed for the immune system and we generally find that modern diets are deficient in all three of these. Magnesium is found in good quantities in sunflower seeds, porridge oats and brown rice. Selenium is found in kidneys and liver, fish and shellfish and whole grains. Zinc is found in oysters, meat, fish and shellfish and hard cheese. If your diet is lacking in meat, fish, shellfish, dairy products and seeds, you may well be lacking in any, or all, of these minerals.

All of the nutritional deficiencies highlighted above can create the environment in which Candida can multiply within us.

How do you know if you have Candida overgrowth?

There are two ways in which you can confirm if you have Candida overgrowth:

1) Have you been exposed to some or many of the *causes* of Candida?

2) Do you have some or many of the *symptoms* of Candida?

1) The causes of Candida are the five listed in the section above:

Immune System: Have you suffered illness in the past two years, which would indicate a weakened immune system?

Carbohydrates: Do you eat processed carbohydrates? (Sugar, white flour, white rice, white pasta, cakes, biscuits, confectionery etc); Do you eat more portions of carbohydrates (including fruit) than fat/protein each day?

Medication: Have you taken antibiotics during childhood?; Have you taken antibiotics during adulthood?; Have you taken birth control pills?; Have you taken hormones in any other form?; Have you taken steroids (e.g. predisone or cortisone)?; Have you ever been pregnant?

Diabetes: Are you diabetic?

Nutritional Deficiency: Do you have any signs of nutritional deficiency such as: white spots on finger nails?; dry flaky skin or brittle hair or nails?; poor hair or skin condition?; muscle aches or general tiredness?; dull, dry eyes?

2) The symptoms of Candida are many and varied. In general, chronic Candida overgrowth can make a person feel very unwell all over. Here are some of the many symptoms that you may be experiencing if you have Candida overgrowth:

Stomach – constipation; diarrhoea; irritable bowel syndrome; stomach distension; bloating, especially after eating; two sets of clothes needed for pre and post eating; indigestion; gas; heartburn.

Head – headaches; dizziness; earaches; blurred vision; flushed cheeks; feeling of 'sleepwalking'; feeling unreal; feeling 'spaced out'.

Women – Pre-Menstrual Tension (PMT); water retention; irregular menstruation; painful breasts; vaginal discharge or itchiness; thrush; cystitis.

Blood Glucose – hungry between meals; irritable or moody before meals; shaky when hungry; faintness when food is not eaten; irregular pulse before and after eating; headaches late morning; waking in the early hours and not being able to get back to sleep; abnormal cravings for sweet foods, bread, alcohol or caffeine; eating sweets increases hunger; excessive appetite; instant sugar 'high' followed by fatigue; chilly feeling after eating.

Mental – anxiety; depression; irritability; lethargy; memory problems; loss of concentration; moodiness; nightmares; mental 'sluggishness'; "*get up and go*" has got up and gone.

Other – athlete's foot; dandruff or other fungal infections; Food Intolerance; dramatic fluctuations in weight from one day to the next; poor circulation; hands and feet sensitive to cold; exhaustion; feeling of being unable to cope; constant fatigue; muscle aches; susceptibility to infection; gasping for breath; sighing often – 'hunger for air'; tightness in chest; chest aches; cramps; yawning easily; insomnia; excessive thirst; easy weight gain; coated tongue; dry skin; hair loss; symptoms worse after consuming yeast or sugary foods; symptoms worse on damp, humid or rainy days.

As you can see, the complaints attributable to Candida are many and varied. If you are feeling very unwell at the moment you may identify with many of the above symptoms and you may be as worried about your general health as you are about your eating habits. However, many readers will be most aware of the sugar handling problems, water retention, fatigue, easy weight gain, dramatic fluctuations in weight, stomach bloating, depression, anxiety and other symptoms common to eating problems. If Candida is left unchecked you could soon develop many of the other symptoms until your health deteriorates to an unprecedented level. Candida does not get better on its own – it gets worse. At the moment you may just be worried about sugar cravings and weight fluctuations but things could get a lot worse.

How does Candida contribute to food cravings/addiction?

Candida is a living organism and every living thing has a natural self-preservation mechanism – we all fight to survive. The yeast living inside us is no exception. The Candida needs processed carbohydrates to feed it. It thrives on a weak immune system. It hates garlic and nutrients as they attack it and kill it off.

If you have Candida overgrowth, you are having a constant battle with your body – you are trying to feel well but the Candida is trying to survive. The things needed for your wellbeing and the Candida's wellbeing are the opposite. When Candida really takes hold you will crave the foods that feed the yeast to ensure it grows and flourishes. If you crave burgers, you may well be craving the ketchup you put on them or the sugar, breadcrumbs and preservatives added to the meat. If you crave salad, it may well be the dressing that you are really after with its vinegar and sugar ingredients. You can pretty much guarantee that you are not craving naked lettuce leaves and plain grilled meat.

You crave the items that feed the yeast, therefore, – all sugary foods, processed carbohydrates, concentrated fruit sugar, yeast and yeast derivatives and vinegary/pickled foods. There is evidence to suggest that eating yeast itself does not feed the yeast, but the consumption of bread and other foods containing yeast generally maintains the environment that the yeast needs to thrive in your body.

There are some great case studies from books on Candida, which give specific examples of the food cravings that Candida sufferers experience. Shirley S Lorenzani writes in her excellent book about Candida driven cravings:

"Every night, at approximately 2am, Dr Jones dragged himself from bed, pulled on a pair of slacks over his pyjamas, and sped to an all-night grocery store. Roaming the aisles like a madman, he threw éclairs, pickles, smoked fish, and ice-cream into the cart. Unable to wait to feast at the kitchen table, he spread the items on the car seat, tore into a couple of wrappers, and began an engorgement that would end when the food did.

Candida overgrowth brings a craving for most of these forbidden (on the anti-Candida diet) foods – not just a preference but a strong virtually insatiable craving. People report dragging themselves out of bed at 2am to go to the all-night grocery."

Shirley S Lorenzani *Candida – a Twentieth Century Disease*

Another excellent book about Candida called *The Yeast Syndrome* is by John Parks Trowbridge and Morton Walker. There is a passage in this book about one of their patients:

"For a long time the woman had suffered with anorexia and bulimia. She dropped from 170 to 140 pounds... her menstrual flow stopped completely when food bingeing alternating with forced vomiting brought her weight down to 115 pounds... constant fatigue and addictive food cravings were additional troubles for Mrs. Bennett...Mrs. Bennett described several weeks of intense sugar cravings that had caused her to gobble down many refined carbohydrates – candy, cake, bread... "

John Parks Trowbridge & Morton Walker *The Yeast Syndrome*.

There are many other references in magazine articles, web pages and books on Candida. It is an absolutely documented fact that people with Candida overgrowth experience addict-like food cravings. People will drive to a grocery store in the middle of the night to feed the cravings and in so doing they will feed the yeast driving the cravings and make the cravings even worse in the future. The more you give into the cravings, the worse the Candida will get and the worse the cravings will get. It really is a vicious circle. The good news is that there is a virtuous circle, which is just as easy to get into, if you can break the vicious circle. The virtuous circle goes something like – you don't give in to the cravings, you fight the yeast with diet and supplements, the cravings get easier, you get stronger, the Candida gets weaker, the cravings get easier and so on. The more you give in to Candida induced cravings the worse they will get – you have to break the cycle and free yourself from the food addiction that is ruining your desire to be slim and probably your overall health and life.

How can you treat Candida?

There are some excellent writers who have focused on Candida such as Leon Chaitow, John Parks Trowbridge & Morton Walker and William G. Crook. There are three main pieces of advice for people suffering from Candida:

1) Starve the Candida overgrowth with diet.

2) Attack the Candida overgrowth with supplements that kill the yeast.

3) Treat the causes so that it doesn't come back.

1) **Starve the Candida**. The dietary advice varies a little but there is a basic diet that all practitioners would advocate – beautifully summed up by Trowbridge & Walker's expression MEVY – Meat/fish, Eggs, Vegetables and Natural Live Yoghurt (NLY). Then the authors vary a little on what other things they allow on top of this. I have tried to summarise the advice from their books in the following table.

In what follows, Trowbridge & Walker recommend that their stage 1 should last three to four weeks; stage 2 may be necessary for three to four months and stage 3 can last for up to two years. If you have severe Candida overgrowth, you may need to avoid foods, as advised in this table, for as long as this. The majority of you should feel substantially better following The Harcombe Diet Phase 1 and then moving cautiously into Phase 2.

	THE YEAST SYNDROME Trowbridge & Walker	CANDIDA ALBICANS Chaitow	THE YEAST CONNECTION Crook
Staples	Meat, fish, eggs, tofu	Meat, fish, eggs, tofu	Meat, fish, eggs, tofu
Vegetables	All veg. & salad except: potatoes, sweet corn, beans, lentils, mushrooms	All veg. & salad except: potatoes, beans, pulses, lentils, chickpeas, mushrooms	All veg. & salad except mushrooms. (Eat starchy vegetables cautiously)
Fruit	None	None for 3-4 weeks	None for 2-3 weeks
Dairy	NLY	NLY	NLY
Grains	None in stage 1. Corn, quinoa & rice in stage 2. Oats, rye & wheat in stage 3	Brown rice, oats, quinoa, whole-wheat bread with no yeast	Barley, corn, millet, oats, rice, wheat (eat all cautiously)
Other	Herbal tea	Herbal tea Nuts in shells Seeds Olive oil	Nuts Seeds Some oils
Key to avoid	Vinegar, mushrooms, yeast, sugar, refined carbohydrates	Vinegar, mushrooms, yeast, sugar, refined carbs, soy sauce, citric acid, MSG, all cheese, nuts not in shells	Vinegar, mushrooms, yeast, sugar, refined carbs, soy sauce, citric acid, MSG, cheeses, melons, dried fruits
Re-introduction of foods	In 4 stages. Some grains in stage 2, most fruits, milk & mushrooms in stage 4	Stay off milk, melons, mushrooms, cheese, bread, vinegar as long as possible	All fruit in moderation, whole grains after a few weeks

2) **Attack the Candida** overgrowth with supplements that kill the yeast. Candida hates all of the following:

- Garlic – scientists have shown that garlic added to colonies of bacteria have ceased the functioning of that bacteria in minutes. Hence garlic is a well known and well-documented antibacterial agent. Garlic has also been shown to be active against yeast and fungi.
- Biotin – research has shown that where a biotin deficiency exists, Candida changes more rapidly from its relatively harmless yeast form to its more dangerous multiplying form. Hence biotin has been shown to be a most useful vitamin in controlling Candida overgrowth.
- Olive oil – contains oleic acid, which prohibits the growth of the yeast in much the same way as biotin.
- Caprylic acid – which comes from coconut oil. You can get user friendly versions of this from some health food shops or from Internet suppliers.
- Lactobacillus Acidophilus – this is one of the major 'friendly' bacteria in our digestive systems and it can, therefore, be used to redress the balance of the gut flora and to fight off the Candida. Again health food shops and Internet suppliers will have this.

3) **Treat the cause** so that it doesn't return. Go back to the 'What causes Candida overgrowth?' section and see where the roots for your problem were:

- A weakened immune system – eat well, drink plenty of water, exercise regularly, don't smoke, drink alcohol in moderation, take time out to do things you enjoy, laugh, socialise, strive for balance. We all know the many things we can do to keep our health optimal and our immune system the strongest it can be.
- Over-consumption of processed carbohydrates – don't go back to consuming lots of sugary, yeasty, vinegary foods once you have got Candida back under control or you will be asking for it to return.

- Medication – steroids, antibiotics, birth control pills, hormones – try to avoid taking any of these if at all possible. Clearly, serious illness requires treatment and unwanted pregnancies are not to be risked, but try to minimise the ingestion of all of the above. Is there an alternative form of contraception? See if you can heal a mild infection with vitamin C and natural remedies before reaching for the antibiotics etc.
- Diabetes – you can still do things to help your situation if diabetes is the factor that has caused your yeast overgrowth. You can manage your carbohydrate intake carefully to reduce the level of glucose in your blood, which may cause yeast overgrowth. Some individuals have been able to reduce the level of insulin they take and some even come off it altogether by following a very low-carbohydrate diet. If you are insulin dependent you must work with your doctor to establish the best eating plan and level of insulin for you. One thing that you can be sure of is that your health can only improve with the elimination of processed carbohydrates from your diet.
- Nutritional deficiency – eat as wide a variety as possible of meat, fish, eggs, dairy products, vegetables and salads and you should have no problem with nutritional deficiency. The most common causes of nutritional deficiency in the developed world are self inflicted – smoking, drinking too much alcohol, dieting and eating processed carbohydrates, leaving little room for more nutritious foods.

What else can I read if I want to know more?

Candida – a Twentieth Century Disease by Shirley Lorenzani (1986)

The Yeast Syndrome by John Parks Trowbridge MD and Morton Walker D.P.M. (1986)

Candida Albicans – Could Yeast be your problem? by Leon Chaitow (1987)

The Yeast Connection by William G. Crook MD (1983)

The Complete Candida Yeast Guidebook by Martin & Rona (2000)

Beat Candida by Gill Jacobs (1990)

Top tips for inspiration

This is worse than Star Wars! There is a parasite inside you, which is demanding to be fed, leading to you feeling dreadful – overweight, spaced out, tired, bloated and hardly able to get through the day. This parasite thrives on sugar, vinegary foods and yeast, as anyone who makes beer or wine will know. The more you feed it, the stronger it gets and the weaker you get.

Don't give this parasite anything it wants. Starve it by depriving it of all the foods it wants and kill it with supplements that it hates. How dare this thing try to take over your body? The good news is that you can devastate it very quickly in the battle. After just five days on a strict anti-Candida diet you can destroy a lot of your Candida overgrowth. You will have cravings like you have never known, in the early stages, and you could experience some quite unpleasant 'die-off' symptoms as you kill the yeast but this should only serve to strengthen your resolve. You may feel temporarily worse but soon you will start feeling quite dramatically better. Even after these first five tough days you could be feeling more energetic, less spaced out, the cravings should have subsided substantially and you will have lost pounds in weight.

Just imagine that every time you put processed carbohydrate or vinegary food in your mouth you are putting petrol into the Candida's tank – you are literally fuelling this parasite that is making your life a misery. Keep this image in your mind every time you have a craving and you will soon rather do anything than feed this monster. Don't see processed carbohydrates as delicious – they are petrol for the enemy. Just visualise bacteria multiplying in your body with every mouthful you eat and this should ease the cravings.

If you don't attack this parasite it will just get stronger and stronger and you will feel weaker and weaker. You have to get it back in control sometime so start straight away before it gets any worse.

Quick summary of Chapter Six

- Candida is a yeast that lives in all of us. It serves no useful purpose. When it gets out of control it can create havoc in our bodies. You have to kill off this parasite before it does any more harm inside your body.

- The main causes of Candida are 1) a weakened immune system, 2) eating things that feed Candida, 3) medication, such as antibiotics and steroids, 4) Diabetes and 5) nutritional deficiency.

- A wide variety of symptoms – physical and psychological – can indicate that Candida is overgrown inside you.

- Candida contributes to food cravings by demanding that you feed it – it loves processed carbohydrates, yeast and sugar in particular. This parasite can produce uncontrollable food cravings as it drives you to feed it so it can grow more and produce even stronger food cravings.

- You can treat it with a three step approach – 1) starve the Candida with your diet 2) attack the Candida overgrowth with supplements like garlic and 3) treat the causes so that it doesn't come back.

Chapter Seven

****

Food Intolerance

What is Food Intolerance?

The definition of 'allergy' is:

*"The condition of reacting adversely to certain substances –
especially food or pollen."*

We should make the distinction at the outset that we are
talking about Food Intolerance and not allergy as defined
above. Food allergy refers to potential fatal reactions to a
substance, such as with nut allergies. If someone has a food
allergy the chances are that they were born with this allergy,
will always have this allergy and it is a very serious condition.
Common allergenic foods include nuts, shellfish, strawberries,
I even know someone violently allergic to kiwis. If a person is
exposed to the food, to which they are allergic, reactions range
from breaking out into a rash, to extreme vomiting/stomach
upset, or even death.

This chapter is *not* about **food allergy**. We are interested in
Food Intolerance, which more generally means having an
intolerance to a particular food or foods. By intolerance we
mean an adverse reaction – not an extreme life threatening
reaction as with food allergy – but any adverse reaction, which
causes the person discomfort. Adverse reactions can include
anything from gastrointestinal disorders to headaches and
reactions which affect the mental state of the person who has
consumed the food.

The following are the most common features of Food
Intolerance (the what, when and how):

What – Food Intolerance develops with repeated overexposure to a particular food. The key words here are 'repeated' and 'overexposure'. It is common for people to become intolerant to foods that they eat a lot of and on a regular basis.

The foods most likely to cause intolerance are, therefore, the ones that are most common. The book *The False Fat Diet*, by Elson M Haas MD & Cameron Stauth, which was written in the United States, says that the most common foods to cause sensitivity are: dairy products; wheat; corn; eggs; soy; peanuts and sugar. (Corn, soy and peanuts are eaten frequently in the USA, but far less so in the UK.)

In Australia the most common Food Intolerances are to milk and wheat. Dr. Brostoff, one of the leading Food Intolerance specialists in the UK, lists the most common foods causing intolerance in the UK as milk and wheat. Dr. Brostoff also noted that for a doctor working in Taiwan, rice and soya beans were the chief culprits. The finger should point at whichever foods are most commonly eaten in the local cuisine.

When – Food Intolerance is not fixed as with food allergy and it can vary over time. People can find themselves susceptible to certain foods at different stages of their lives. For example, someone suffering from stress can develop intolerance to a food that they are consuming a lot of at the time and then be able to eat the food again in moderation at other times in their life. Pregnant women sometimes develop a sensitivity to a particular food that disappears after childbirth.

The other interesting aspect of Food Intolerance, related to time, is that the adverse reaction is not immediate as with food allergy. For example, a person can eat a food to which they are intolerant and develop symptoms over the next twenty-four to forty-eight hours. When I had a wheat intolerance, I used to develop an upset stomach within hours and then the day after I felt completely exhausted and my muscles ached, as if I had run a marathon. This makes the identification of Food Intolerance all the more difficult as often many other foods have been eaten since the offending food, so it is difficult to pin-point the exact food, or foods, which have caused the reaction.

How – The offending food produces a state of wellbeing ranging from a slight mood change to an almost manic state of euphoria. This is when the addictive aspect of Food Intolerance takes hold. Gradually more and more of the offending food is needed to produce the state of wellbeing previously provided by a normal portion of the food. At this stage necessity is starting to replace desire. There is a need for the food and withdrawal symptoms will arise if the food is not eaten. For example, if you find that you get a headache mid-morning, if you don't have your usual breakfast, there may well be something that you are consuming at breakfast to which you have become intolerant.

What causes Food Intolerance?

The clue is in the text above – 'repeated' and 'overexposure'. It is estimated that we rely on as few as a dozen foods on a daily basis and that almost all of these will come from the milk, sugar and wheat food families. We eat toast or cereal for breakfast with milk (milk, sugar and wheat). We often have sugary snacks, and milk in tea and coffee, throughout the day (milk, sugar and wheat). We may have pasta, sandwiches or pizza for main meals (wheat and often milk and sugar again). If we have a salad, meat or fish, we may well have wheat or dairy with it, such as cheese, bread or crisp breads and so on. With repeated overexposure to any food, our bodies can become intolerant to this food and we will start to experience withdrawal symptoms if we don't have the food (this is when we are officially addicted to the food and the cravings for the food will be making us overeat).

How do you know if you are affected by Food Intolerance?

As with Candida the range of symptoms related to Food Intolerance are many and varied. There are also remarkable overlaps, which is why, so often, people with extreme cravings and weight problems are suffering from both conditions. The complaints include:

Stomach – constipation; diarrhoea; irritable bowel syndrome; stomach distension; bloating, especially after eating; two sets of clothes needed for pre and post eating; indigestion; gas; heartburn.

Head – headaches; dizziness; flushed cheeks; feeling of 'sleepwalking'; feeling unreal; feeling 'spaced out'.

Women – PMT; water retention; irregular menstruation.

Blood Glucose – hungry between meals; irritable or moody before meals; shaky when hungry; faintness when food is not eaten; irregular pulse before and after eating; headaches late morning; waking in the early hours and not being able to get back to sleep; abnormal cravings for sweets or caffeine; eating sweets increases hunger; excessive appetite; instant sugar 'high' followed by fatigue; chilly feeling after eating.

Mental – anxiety; depression; irritability; lethargy; memory problems; loss of concentration; moodiness; nightmares; mental 'sluggishness'; reduced 'get up and go'.

Other symptoms – dramatic fluctuations in weight from one day to the next; exhaustion; feeling of being unable to cope; constant fatigue; muscle aches; susceptibility to infection; gasping for breath; sighing often – 'hunger for air'; chest aches; cramps; excessive thirst; easy weight gain; coated tongue; dry skin; itchiness/rashes.

Dr. Brostoff uses a nice phrase which is "thick note syndrome." Where doctors see a medical file which is thick and full of varied and seemingly unconnected complaints, they would be well advised to ask the person what they are eating.

How does Food Intolerance contribute to food cravings/addiction?

The real irony is that the foods to which you are intolerant are the foods that you crave. Just as the drug addict or smoker craves their fix, so you crave the substances that are causing you harm. It starts off with a particular food or drink that you consume on regular occasions. The most common offenders are dairy products and wheat as we have them in so many different forms during the day. Any substance that we eat daily can start to cause problems and those we eat regularly, several times a day, are the chief suspects. It takes three to four days for a digested substance to pass through our bodies, so we can overload our bodies with one particular substance if we eat it daily or even more often.

Our bodies then literally become 'intolerant' to the food – i.e. they can't cope with any more of it. You would think that we would shun a food if we had become intolerant to it but in fact the addiction that goes with Food Intolerance actually means that the opposite happens. If we remember back to the definition of addiction, we go through these stages with Food Intolerance:

1) We start with an uncontrollable craving.

2) We then need more and more of the offending substance in order to get the same 'high'.

3) We develop physical and/or psychological dependence.

4) We suffer the adverse effects.

If you want to know what you are intolerant to, simply ask yourself honestly the food(s) you would least like to give up. If you cannot imagine life without bread or cereal you should suspect wheat. If you can't face a day without eggs in any form (e.g. some pasta is egg based) then eggs could be your problem. It is so cruel but the foods that we don't crave – those we could take or leave – are the foods that we need to keep in our diets. However, even these we need to eat in moderation and irregularly as most foods can become a problem if we have repeated overexposure.

The following extracts from books on Food Intolerance capture the addictive nature of Food Intolerance beautifully:

"Specific allergic adaptation to foods and chemicals is an addiction as devastating as addiction to tobacco or drugs. In my opinion, only heroin or morphine addiction are more potent and destructive than severe food addiction, which I would put on a par with alcoholism."

Dr. Richard Mackarness *Not all in the mind.*

"Bread is another good example of an addictive allergy. Some individuals just cannot go without bread, even for a day – toast for breakfast, sandwiches for lunch, bread for dinner. The standard reaction to the suggestion of 'no more bread' is the statement 'what is there left to eat?'. This type of person can quite easily consume up to one loaf of bread a day and it is usual to find them consuming half a loaf."

"These addictive foods are always over-consumed and at frequent intervals. If you miss eating them you will start to feel bad. When you miss having your regular fix you start to have withdrawal symptoms just like a drug addict. Your body starts rebelling against the removal of the food on which it has come to depend."

Robert Buist *Food Intolerance.*

"...we reach a stage of addiction : the patient craves the food and wants to eat it often, even to binge the food. The reason is that by this stage, ironically, the patient gets the symptoms only if he or she doesn't eat the food."

Dr. Keith Mumby *The Allergy Handbook.*

"Food addiction differs only in degree of severity from a drug addiction."

"The American humorist Don Marquis once said that 'ours is a world where people don't know what they want and are willing to go through hell to get it.' This is a good description of the food addict, who doesn't know the exact nature of the food he craves, but is willing to eat compulsively, to the point of addiction, in order to get it."

In reference to a clinic patient: "I've reached the point where I am afraid to eat any longer. Once I start eating, I feel as if I simply cannot stop."

Discussing a food addict: "He may wake up in the middle of the night and help himself to more food. Sometimes family members will joke that he seems to be addicted to sweets, cheese, steak, or whatever is his favourite treat. If only they knew how right they are!"

Theron Randolph & Ralph Moss *Allergies – Your Hidden Enemy*.

"Millions of men, women and children suffer from the addictive form of food allergy... Obese people are living testaments to the strength of food addiction... The foods to which the compulsive eater has an addictive allergy are never skipped, and eating for the relief of food-related withdrawal symptoms may become the obese person's interest in life... Progressive overweight develops as the advancing stage of allergic food addiction requires increasing doses of the specific food(s) to satisfy the craving... the compulsive eater is not overwhelmed with emotional problems or an unfulfilled need for love that requires oral gratification. He is a chronic foodaholic with a serious but easily diagnosable nonpsychological ailment."

Dr. Marshall Mandell & Lynne Scanlon *5-Day Allergy Relief System*.

"Food reactions are the single most common cause of the cravings that destroy diets. These cravings, which are far harder to resist than mere hunger, are similar to the physical urges experienced by alcoholics or cigarette smokers."

Elson M Haas MD & Cameron Stauth *The False Fat Diet*.

All of these passages confirm why you overeat – when all you want is to be slim. One of the reasons is almost certainly that you are intolerant to some foods. The intolerance will drive addict-like cravings, which is why you feel you have no control over your eating whatsoever.

How can you treat Food Intolerance?

To regain control you need to identify those foods to which you are intolerant and eliminate them from your diet. You will go through intense withdrawal symptoms while you do this but the good news is that these should last fewer than five days – just a bit more than the time it takes for a substance to pass through your body completely. You will then find that, if you eat the offending food after avoiding it for some time, you may experience extreme and sudden reactions, which is your body's way of confirming that this food is not good for you.

The key steps to treating Food Intolerance are, therefore, quite simple – find out what is causing you problems and stop eating it. Don't get depressed thinking you are about to give up some foods for life. Unlike food allergy, which remains for a life-time, Food Intolerance does come and go over time. Hence you could find yourself intolerant to, say, dairy products, during a stressful period of your life when your immune system is particularly low and you may find you can tolerate dairy products again when your health is better. Many people find that they can re-introduce foods to which they have been intolerant in time, when their immunity has recovered, but only on an infrequent basis. In other words, you will probably find that you can return to consuming any food or drink, in time, but you are likely to find that your symptoms and cravings reappear quite quickly as soon as you eat the substance too much or too often.

Step 1 – Identify the foods

The best way to identify the foods to which you are intolerant is to keep a food diary and test individual foods carefully and one at a time. Here are the practical steps to take:

- You can start with some educated guesses as to what your problem foods are likely to be. The foods that you crave are the ones that are most likely to be causing you problems.

Anything that you eat often and in large, or increasing, quantities should be suspected. Anything that you really can't imagine *not* eating is to be suspected.

- You must start a food diary, as changes can be subtle over time and it may be that you need to compare diary entries days or weeks apart to notice how far you have progressed. However, the outcome could also be quite dramatic and not at all subtle. Buy a notebook and write down everything you eat and how you feel afterwards. This alone may establish a pattern. For example, if after every entry with bread, pasta, cakes or biscuits you record that you experience bloating and stomach problems, you can start to suspect wheat as a problem.
- When you have started recording what you eat and how it makes you feel you can try to cut out the foods that you suspect and again there are a number of ways in which you can do this. You can keep your eating patterns as close to your normal eating as possible and just cut out foods that you suspect or, at the other extreme, you can start a very limited diet and re-introduce foods from there. This is when we move onto Step 2.

Step 2 – Stop eating them

When you move onto food elimination it is really important to keep that food diary going to notice any changes that do occur. Phase 1 has already been designed to be the perfect diet to overcome Food Intolerance (along with Candida and Hypoglycaemia at the same time). So start Phase 1 and be prepared to avoid the foods, which you have identified in Step 1 as a problem for you, for longer than five days.

When you do re-introduce foods, the food diary becomes more important than ever, as you will need this to confirm the foods that are problems for you personally.

There are two ways in which the avoidance of foods can help identify and, therefore, treat Food Intolerance. It may sound simple and obvious but when you stop eating a problem food you should feel better and when you start eating a

114

problem food again you should feel worse. The slight complication is that *initially*, when you first stop eating an offending food, you may feel a lot worse and your cravings could be as bad as ever.

Remember that you are craving food because you are trying to avoid the withdrawal symptoms that you get when you don't have the food to which you are intolerant. Hence, when you first stop eating the problem food, the withdrawal symptoms are going to come out in force. This is where the food diary will really help as you may record feeling exhausted, lethargic and depressed and with unbearable cravings for one to five days. However, after these first few days you should feel much better. If you avoid an offending food for a few days or weeks and then go back to eating it you can suffer quite dramatic bad symptoms. However, if you avoid an offending food for a long period of time, such as months or years, you could equally find that you have no problems with the food that previously caused you trouble.

Food Intolerance is quite a complex and sensitive area and it reflects your overall wellbeing at any one time, so it will change as you do. A food diary will really help to show what causes immediate problems (e.g. cravings, bloating) and what causes problems up to a day after (stomach upset, fatigue). You need to become highly tuned in to what you eat and how it makes you feel.

Here are the practical tips for re-introducing foods to confirm foods that you suspect are causing you problems and/or to give other foods the all clear:

- Eat single foods not processed foods. If you react badly to a cake, you won't know if sugar, wheat, eggs or dairy products are your problem as they are all in a cake. To test each substance you need to eat it on its own, e.g. to test wheat, eat shredded wheat (100% whole-wheat) on its own; to test dairy products, try milk on its own; to test eggs, eat eggs on their own etc.

- Eat one food at a time – one of the best ways to test foods is to avoid them for at least five days (so that there are no traces of them in your system) and then re-introduce them one by one and check for symptoms. e.g. have wheat on its own for breakfast, have only eggs for lunch and then only corn for dinner. As this is very restrictive it can be made easier by mixing one food to be tested with foods that you know don't cause you a problem. It is rare for people to be intolerant to meat, fish and vegetables so have these at each meal with just one other food that you are testing at that meal. If you suffer symptoms, you can then be pretty sure which food has caused the problems.
- Eat food a few hours apart – don't test one food within four hours of another as the symptoms may take time to show and you could mistakenly think that the second food has caused the problem.
- Assume that the foods you most crave and would most miss are the ones causing you problems. If there are any foods that you never crave, and could happily live without, sadly these are the ones that you need to have in your eating plan until your Food Intolerance is brought under control.

In summary, to treat Food Intolerance you need to identify the food(s) to which you are intolerant and eliminate them for as long as necessary. The complications are in the detail – how long is necessary? How do you know which foods? I hope that the above section has suggested a number of ways in which you can identify your own problem foods, how you can cut them out of your diet and how you can re-introduce them to test them for confirmation. The final stage, once your immunity and health is restored, is to eat as wide a variety of food as possible, trying not to eat any food every day and keeping a lookout for any cravings and other symptoms which could indicate that Food Intolerance has returned.

What else can I read if I want to know more?

Food Intolerance – What it is & How to cope with it by Robert Buist (1984)

5-day Allergy Relief System by Dr. Marshall Mandell and Lynne Scanlon (1979)

The Allergy Handbook by Dr. Keith Mumby (1988)

Allergies – Your Hidden Enemy? by Theron Randolph MD & Ralph W. Moss PhD (1981)

Not all in the Mind by Dr. Richard Mackarness (1976)

The False Fat Diet by Elson Haas & Cameron Stauth (2001)

The Complete Guide to Food Allergy and Intolerance by Dr. Jonathan Brostoff & Linda Gamlin (1989)

Top tips for inspiration

This is one of the easiest conditions to address. Unlike Candida, which can take weeks to get under control, you can stop the cravings which follow from Food Intolerance in a maximum of five days. It takes fewer than five days for the substance causing you problems to have cleared itself from your body and there will then be no reason for you to crave that substance any longer. You are likely to have tough withdrawal symptoms for the first few days, but then you will feel better than you have done for ages – mentally more alert, more energetic and clear headed.

Just think – you can be free from your Food Intolerance cravings in just five days. You can be rid of that puffy, red face that greets you each morning. You can be free from stomach bloating and digestive problems that are caused by intolerance to a particular food.

One of the best inspirational tips is that you could lose pounds as soon as you stop eating a food to which you are intolerant. Food Intolerance leads to dramatic water retention. When you stop eating a food that is causing you problems you are likely to lose pounds very quickly indeed and you will find that your rings, shoes and clothes fit better than ever before.

Quick summary of Chapter Seven

- Food *allergy* is the condition of reacting badly to certain substances – like nuts or strawberries. It can be life threatening. It is not what this chapter is about.

- Food *Intolerance* is the condition of being intolerant to a particular food or foods. It is not life threatening, but it can make you feel quite unwell in a variety of ways.

- The key cause of Food Intolerance is repeated overexposure to a certain food – having too much of it and too often.

- The symptoms of Food Intolerance are many and varied and include physical, as well as psychological, complaints.

- Food Intolerance leads to food cravings because you ironically crave the foods to which you are intolerant. A sure sign of Food Intolerance is having a substance that you crave uncontrollably and try to eat as often as possible.

- You treat Food Intolerance quite simply by not eating the foods to which you are intolerant. You probably won't have to avoid them forever as, when your immune system is stronger, you may well be able to tolerate them again.

Chapter Eight

****

Hypoglycaemia

What is Hypoglycaemia?

Hypoglycaemia is literally a Greek translation from "*hypo*" meaning 'under', "*glykis*" meaning 'sweet' and "*emia*" meaning 'in the blood together'. The three bits all put together mean low blood glucose. (It is sometimes known as hyperinsulinism, as the opposite of low blood glucose is excessive insulin). It follows that the causes of Hypoglycaemia are factors that trigger the pancreas to release insulin in response to a rise in blood glucose level. Sugar and processed carbohydrates are the main offenders but caffeine, allergic substances, stress and alcohol may all prompt a similar response.

What diabetes can teach us about Hypoglycaemia

We defined diabetes in Chapter Four and the definition is in the Glossary at the back of this book for convenience.

In 1924, during the investigation of diabetes and the development of insulin, it was observed by Dr. Seale Harris that non-diabetic people had reactions similar to diabetics who had taken too much insulin. A paper on 'hyperinsulinism' was published in the Journal of the American Medical Association. Further research by Harris found that Hypoglycaemia, as the condition became known, was the result of a defect in the blood glucose regulating system. Subsequent research has shown how crucial the blood glucose balance is for a healthy body and mind and yet, almost a century after the initial studies, many doctors believe that millions of people are still undiagnosed as hypoglycaemic. Instead they are labelled neurotic, anxious, depressed, fatigued, stressed, anti-social and moody. They may also be labelled alcoholic or bulimic if they suffer from compulsive drinking and eating, as do many hypoglycaemics.

If a diabetic takes too much insulin the following symptoms may arise – weakness, tremors, clammy hands, sweating, fainting, blackouts, hunger, thirst, mental confusion, exhaustion, irritability and many other symptoms. As the brain and central nervous system rely on stable and adequate supplies of blood glucose for normal function, the most dramatic symptoms of Hypoglycaemia are shown in the emotional and mental state of a person. Many psychiatric disorders can be prompted by low blood glucose – amnesia, negativism, personality changes, maniacal behaviour, emotional instability and delirium. Diabetics who have their insulin injection and then delay their meal, or eat too little relative to the amount of insulin injected, can display quite alarming symptoms. In the extreme they can lapse into a coma and die.

I have witnessed a diabetic in a state of low blood glucose after taking too much insulin relative to food intake one evening. He had a total lack of awareness and co-ordination to the extent that, when his girlfriend suggested that he should put his shoes on to leave, he just nodded 'yes' and didn't move. The request was repeated on several occasions until those around him realised that he could not register what his shoes were, let alone whether or not he had them on, and how to put them on if they were not already on. He was extremely withdrawn, distant and completely dopey. (Incidentally this diabetic was a 26 year old Cambridge graduate). The apathetic, confused, disorientated 'overeater' who sits for hours staring at the floor or ceiling after a binge may be suffering from similar problems with blood glucose.

In a non-diabetic person, as food is eaten, the pancreas releases insulin to compensate for the rise in blood glucose that occurs as food is ingested. Thus a key role of the pancreas is to ensure that glucose balance is maintained with no glucose leaving the body as a waste product.

This function performed by the pancreas is one of the most delicate balancing operations performed by the body and there is increasing evidence that the modern western diet is disturbing this mechanism. Since man first walked upright, an estimated 3.5 million years ago, we ate whatever animals we could hunt and vegetation, fruits, nuts and seeds as seasonally and geographically available. Grains and dairy products were introduced to the human diet approximately 10,000 years ago, which is no time at all in terms of evolution. The current consumption of cakes, sweets, biscuits, ice cream, sugary drinks and so on is unprecedented throughout history. Furthermore, sugar is found in almost all modern consumer foods from cereal to yoghurt and from baked beans to prepared salads.

Medical opinion is divided on the subject of the prevalence of disturbed carbohydrate tolerance or 'Reactive Hypoglycaemia' as a result of the typical western diet. However, it cannot be disputed that blood glucose will remain more stable, and the pancreas will have to react less, on a diet of meat and vegetables than on a diet of sugar and carbohydrates. Given this undisputable fact and given the evidence that we have of the impact of blood glucose level on the body and mind, it remains a complete mystery to me why so many doctors dismiss the notion of Hypoglycaemia and treat people with anti-depressants and other drugs before trying a change in diet.

On a diet of fat/protein and vegetables, blood glucose remains well balanced and quite stable whereas on a diet of sugar and carbohydrates the pancreas is overworked at regular intervals and the blood glucose level peaks and troughs with the amplitude of a wave frequency motion. If you had a very sophisticated pair of scales, capable of weighing individual grains of rice, would you put a sack of potatoes on them? This is effectively what you are doing to your body if you eat carbohydrates at regular intervals and your tolerance for them is anything less than perfect.

If we apply the theory of Hypoglycaemia to eating disorders, consider the overeater who tries to starve for a day and becomes restless, crabby, irritable, depressed and sometimes emotionally unstable. The overeater then breaks their fast with, say, a confectionery bar and becomes hyperactive, manic, bubbly, talkative and alert for probably no more than two hours before the depression and emotional instability returns. The psychological theory suggests that the overeater is depressed and unstable during the fast because they are not blotting out emotional problems by eating. When they eat they feel temporary relief and then feel guilty afterwards. Undoubtedly the overeater does feel guilty after eating, but it may be low blood glucose causing the symptoms of depression and instability rather than fundamental psychological problems. This seems to have been overlooked by doctors and psychologists to date.

Fluctuations in blood glucose are as important to Hypoglycaemia as the *actual* level of blood glucose. If the blood glucose level falls *rapidly* below normal, symptoms include sweating, weakness, hunger, rapid beating of the heart and a feeling of fear or anxiety. If the blood glucose level falls *slowly* over a period of time, a person may suffer headaches, blurred vision, mental confusion, crabbiness, irritability and incoherent speech. Then, if this fall is sustained for a period of hours, the symptoms may include outburst of temper, extreme depression, sleepiness, restlessness, negativism, emotional instability, manic behaviour and general personality disorders.

The impact of fluctuations in blood glucose levels will also resonate with any overeater who starves and binges. As the fast starts, the blood glucose level falls slowly and the person becomes confused and unable to concentrate. Reactions slow down, memory and mechanical ability suffer and headaches may be extremely unpleasant ('hunger headaches'). The overeater then binges and their blood glucose level rises rapidly and then falls rapidly as insulin is released in compensation. This rapid fall in the blood glucose level prompts hunger, weakness and a feeling of profound anxiety.

This may not be simply anxiety about having binged, but general anxiety caused by Hypoglycaemia.

What causes Hypoglycaemia?

The short answer is - our modern diet. The key cause of Hypoglycaemia is the over consumption of carbohydrates, especially processed ones. We wouldn't try to run our car on the kind of rubbish we put into our own bodies. Putting diesel in a petrol car will grind it to a halt pretty quickly. We do much worse than this, to our far more sophisticated bodies on a daily, if not hourly, basis.

The pancreas is there to help us digest food and to ensure that our blood glucose level remains stable. Without the hormone insulin, which the pancreas produces, we would die. It is as simple as that. The pancreas detects what a person has eaten and releases the appropriate amount of insulin to maintain a healthy blood glucose level. When we eat in the way our ancestors did, the mechanism works well. When we eat meat, fish and plain vegetables our body releases hardly any insulin and our blood glucose level remains stable.

When we drink a carton of apple juice our pancreas thinks we have eaten, say, twenty apples and releases the appropriate amount of insulin for twenty apples. When we eat a confectionery bar, I dread to think what the pancreas thinks it is trying to cope with. What we do know is that the pancreas releases a significant amount of insulin to cope with the sugar onslaught.

When we eat anything other than the whole food, our bodies can release too much insulin. This then lowers our blood glucose to below the level it was before we ate the food. Let us see this in a diagram, as it is critical to understand the peaks and troughs of blood glucose levels, which can be induced by eating processed food. You will be able to see a key driver for food cravings as we do this.

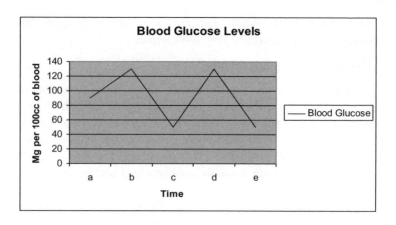

a) In the diagram above, at position 'a' your blood glucose level is stable at approximately 90mg per 100cc of blood.

b) You then eat a confectionery bar and at position 'b' your blood glucose level rises instantly (this is the sugar high/energy high that you experience).

c) Your pancreas then releases insulin to cope with the many pieces of fruit or equivalent sweetness that it thinks you have just eaten and at position 'c' your blood glucose level drops below where it was before you ate the confectionery.

d) This is when your body cries out to be fed and, if you reach for more confectionery, your blood glucose level will shoot back up again as at position 'd'.

e) More insulin will be released and your blood glucose level will then fall below normal levels again, as shown at position 'e', as too much insulin has been released to cope with the second confectionery bar.

When your blood glucose level drops below approximately 65mg per 100cc of blood, your cravings for food will be huge as your body is literally in danger mode. Your blood glucose has dropped to a level which is detrimental to your health and your body will try to do anything to get you to eat to raise your blood glucose level back to normal. If you have a banana or a similar whole carbohydrate you have a reasonable chance of stabilising your blood glucose level. However, if you reach for another confectionery bar you will start the cycle all over again.

This is why once you start eating sweet foods (sweets, ice cream, chocolate, biscuits, cakes etc) you can't stop. It is so much easier not to have chocolate at all than it is to try to eat a limited amount – this really is like asking an alcoholic to have one drink and no more.

This is also why you may find it easier to eat nothing, rather than to try to eat a small amount. When you 'starve' (don't eat) your blood glucose level is low, but at least it is stable. Hence, cravings are actually easier to control when you eat nothing.

The state of Hypoglycaemia can be brought on temporarily and quickly by consuming processed carbohydrates. When we say that someone has Hypoglycaemia what we are really saying is that their pancreas/insulin releasing mechanism is out of balance and that they are constantly in a state of high or low blood glucose. They are rarely at a nice, even, steady level of blood glucose. They swing from one extreme to the other and suffer the energy highs and lows that go with it. This is almost certainly as a result of long term consumption of processed carbohydrates.

Some people do seem to be able to eat processed carbohydrates and 'get away with it'. Their bodies don't seem to release too much insulin, which suggests that some people may be more susceptible to Hypoglycaemia than others. However, in the majority of people, prolonged consumption of processed carbohydrates is likely to cause Hypoglycaemia. In some people it even leads to diabetes. Type 2 diabetes is almost always preceded by Hypoglycaemia (often people did not know that they were suffering from Hypoglycaemia before they were diagnosed as diabetic). Some people's pancreases go from producing too much insulin to not producing enough, or any at all, which is the definition of diabetes.

Diabetes and Hypoglycaemia can both be greatly helped by following an eating plan which contains no processed carbohydrates whatsoever. Eating processed carbohydrates can be a cause of both Hypoglycaemia and type 2 diabetes.

How do you know if you are affected by Hypoglycaemia?

Hypoglycaemia can be diagnosed with a glucose tolerance test, which involves a series of blood tests being taken, after a glucose drink has been drunk, to measure the person's tolerance for sugar. This test is rarely performed at the suggestion of a doctor and it may be difficult to persuade your doctor to refer you for one. The perfectly acceptable alternative is to try the eating plan for Hypoglycaemia and keep a food diary to notice if your symptoms improve or disappear altogether.

If you follow a low-carbohydrate diet for a period of time and your symptoms improve considerably you can be pretty certain that Hypoglycaemia has been a problem for you. One of the best tests, much more readily available than a glucose tolerance test, is to follow the Phase 1 eating plan in this book for five days. If you have stable energy levels, a clear head and your other symptoms of Hypoglycaemia have subsided then you can be sure that Hypoglycaemia was a problem for you.

The symptoms of Hypoglycaemia include the following:

Head – headaches; dizziness; blurred vision; feeling of 'sleepwalking'; feeling unreal; feeling 'spaced out'.

Women – PMT.

Blood Glucose – hungry between meals; irritable or moody before meals; shaky when hungry; faintness when food is not eaten; irregular pulse before and after eating; headaches late morning; waking in the early hours and not being able to get back to sleep; abnormal cravings for sweets or caffeine; eating sweets increases hunger; excessive appetite; instant sugar 'high' followed by fatigue; chilly feeling after eating.

Mental – anxiety; depression; irritability; lethargy; memory problems; loss of concentration; moodiness; nightmares; mental 'sluggishness'; "*get up and go*" has got up and gone.

126

Other – dramatic fluctuations in weight from one day to the next; exhaustion; feeling of being unable to cope; constant fatigue; excessive thirst; easy weight gain.

How does Hypoglycaemia cause food cravings/addiction?

This is a really simple one. As soon as your blood glucose level falls below normal your body will cry out for food. It will crave anything, but most likely sweet foods, to get your blood glucose level back up again. When your hands are shaking, you feel a bit sweaty, a bit light headed or even faint in extreme cases, this is your body begging you to eat. You reach for a confectionery bar and immediately feel better, almost euphoric, as your blood glucose level shoots up. However, this is another substance alien to your pancreas so your body overproduces insulin, your blood glucose level falls below normal again and the cravings continue.

This is exactly why once you start bingeing you can't stop – because your blood glucose level swings from high to below normal and as soon as it is below normal you cannot resist food so you eat and it shoots back up to high again. It is a vicious circle that so many of us go through several times a day.

How can you treat Hypoglycaemia?

This is pretty simple too – stop eating processed carbohydrates and manage carbohydrate intake generally - even natural carbohydrates. Try Phase 1 for a few days to confirm the diagnosis and to see just how well you can feel. Then continue to eat only *unprocessed* (wholemeal) carbohydrates as you progress into Phase 2.

Some of you will need to manage carbohydrate intake more carefully than others. If you have many of the listed symptoms of Hypoglycaemia and know that you are very sensitive to carbohydrates, the more fat meals that you have in Phase 2 and the fewer carb meals, the better this will be for your weight and health.

What else can I read if I want to know more?

Hypoglycaemia – The Disease your Doctor Won't Treat by Saunders & Ross (1980)

Low Blood glucose (Hypoglycaemia) The twentieth century Epidemic? by Martin L Budd (1983)

New low blood sugar & you by Carlton Fredericks (1985)

Top tips for inspiration

This condition is the most serious of all three. Candida can make you feel really ill but it is not life threatening. Food Intolerance, similarly, can make you feel most unwell but it is food *allergy* that is life threatening, not Food *Intolerance*. Hypoglycaemia is potentially very serious. It can lead to diabetes, which is the fourth leading cause of death in most developed countries, third in the USA. At the very least, Hypoglycaemia is your body's way of telling you that something is wrong. It is telling you that your pancreas cannot cope with what you are putting into your body and your pancreas is a vital organ for health and wellbeing.

If you care at all about your health, if the thought of possibly becoming diabetic and injecting insulin once or twice a day frightens you, then take this early warning very seriously.

You have got a highly sensitive balancing system in your body and you are ruining it day by day, hour by hour. You may as well take a set of laboratory scales, capable of weighing a feather, and throw a brick on them.

This is not just about weight – your whole health and body functions are at stake here. You simply must start being kind to your body by giving it foods to nourish it rather than bombarding it with junk.

Quick summary of Chapter Eight

- Hypoglycaemia literally means low blood glucose.

- Hypoglycaemia is primarily caused by the over-consumption of carbohydrates. Some people appear to be more susceptible to it than others, but Hypoglycaemia is now believed to be very widespread.

- The symptoms of Hypoglycaemia are many and varied and include physical as well as psychological complaints.

- Hypoglycaemia leads to food cravings because when your blood glucose level falls below normal, as a result of too much insulin being released, your body will beg you to eat to raise your blood glucose level again. If you eat something else that will result in too much insulin being produced (another carbohydrate), your blood glucose level will fall below normal again and you will be in a vicious cycle of food craving.

- You treat Hypoglycaemia quite simply by not eating processed carbohydrates specifically and managing carbohydrate intake generally. Some people find that they need to limit all carbohydrates, until their insulin mechanism retunes, but usually people can eat wholemeal carbohydrates safely.

Part Three

****

Postscript: Completing the jigsaw

Chapter Three explained how calorie counting/eating less leads directly and indirectly to the three conditions that cause insatiable food cravings: Candida, Food Intolerance and Hypoglycaemia. This makes for the ironic situation that the most likely cause of food cravings is dieting.

However, there are some non-food/dieting routes to food cravings and we should capture these before moving on.

The key outcomes that we need to avoid are: food cravings; overeating; overproduction of insulin (the fattening hormone) and weight gain.

The three conditions that can lead to all of these outcomes are: Candida, Food Intolerance and Hypoglycaemia.

The main causes of the three conditions and, in some cases, direct causes of the outcomes, are both food related and non-food related. The food related causes are: calorie counting; eating a limited variety of foods and a high carbohydrate consumption. Dieting, as we saw in Chapter Three, leads us to eat a limited variety of high carbohydrate foods continually as we try to get the 'biggest bang' for our 'dieting buck'.

The key non-food related causes of the three conditions are: medication; stress and having a weakened immune system. Let us look at these three in turn so that we can ensure that we have all causes of food cravings covered:

CAUSES	Food related: Calorie Counting; Eating a limited variety of food; High carbohydrate consumption. Non-food related: Medication Stress; A weakened immune system.
CONDITIONS	Candida Food Intolerance Hypoglycaemia
OUTCOMES	Food cravings; Overeating; Overproduction of insulin (the fattening hormone); Weight gain.

Medication

For many people medication is the start of the vicious spiral downwards. Frequent doses of antibiotics or being on the contraceptive pill can create the right environment for Candida to proliferate. Candida causes cravings directly. Medication can also weaken the natural immune system giving rise to further Candida overgrowth, Food Intolerance and/or Hypoglycaemia. There is a bit of chicken and egg going on here as people generally take antibiotics because they have an infection, which can be indicative of a weakened immune system, but then the medication may weaken the immune system further.

The vicious cycle just needs one route in and then the problems of cravings, weakened immune system, high consumption of carbohydrates, Candida, Food Intolerance and Hypoglycaemia all feed off each other in an explosive way.

The route in is often calorie counting or medication but it can be stress…

Stress

Stress is the second major causal factor that can start off all of our problems with food and cravings. Stress has a lot to do with the way we eat in the modern world. Our busy lives lead us to eat on the run and grab convenience and fast foods rather than taking the time to prepare fresh vegetable dishes and cook some fish or meat. When we do eat protein it is often low-fat cheese in a sandwich, or burger meat in a bun, or fish in breadcrumbs – we so rarely eat whole foods, simply cooked with no additives or other extras.

Stress also directly affects our blood glucose level as it has been shown that the fright, flight, fight mechanism, which helped cave people get out of dangerous situations, is still present in us today. Our adrenalin is raised not by charging animals or angry tribes, but by traffic queues and rows with our partners or children. Any adrenalin rush has been shown to impact our blood glucose level – even caffeine, which has no calories or carbohydrates, has been shown to impact our blood glucose level as it acts as a stimulant.

Hence the message here is that we are upsetting our blood glucose level throughout the day – not just with the food and drink that we consume, but with caffeine and our stress levels and the way our adrenal glands still work in modern life.

Stress can also lead us to take medication, which can weaken our immune system and then set us off into the vicious circle of causes, conditions, cravings and overeating.

Stress often leads to a high consumption of carbohydrates as we turn to food for comfort. There is a medical logic for this as carbohydrates stimulate production of a substance called serotonin, which has been shown to have an impact on our moods. Hence we are trying to help our bodies when we reach for carbohydrates in times of stress. The trouble is that processed carbohydrates upset our blood glucose balance and general health even further and we then end up in the vicious spiral downwards.

Weakened immune system

A weakened immune system can lead to:

- Candida, as it creates the environment for the yeast to multiply,
- Food Intolerance, as our bodies are more susceptible to adverse reactions to common foods,
- Hypoglycaemia, as our general health is likely to impact our blood glucose level and stability.

A weakened immune system can also lead us to take medication for infections or other health problems and this can then keep the vicious circle going.

To keep reinforcing how interactive all these causes and conditions are, calorie counting leads to a weakened immune system, as we quite literally take in less fuel than we need to sustain ourselves and our bodies are, therefore, deprived of nutrients that they need for optimal health.

Calorie counting also leads us to eat a far more restricted variety of foods, as we avoid high calorie foods in favour of low calorie alternatives. This directly leads to Food Intolerance, as we tend to eat the same foods on a regular basis. This also leads to nutritional deficiency, as the best way to guarantee that we eat all the nutrients that we need is to eat a varied diet and one rich in natural fats from meat, fish, eggs and dairy products. The foods that we generally opt for on low calorie diets also tend to be those that feed Candida overgrowth – fruits, vinegary salads, crisp breads and so on and this, in turn, can weaken our immune system, as Candida takes hold.

Food Intolerance drives us to crave carbohydrates and Hypoglycaemia also has us favouring carbohydrates over salmon and green beans. Every time we opt for low fat, high carbohydrate alternatives to real food we further weaken our immune system as we miss out on optimal nutrition.

Piecing the jigsaw together

We can, therefore, see how completely interrelated a number of factors are and how all of them lead to food cravings and overeating and hence overweight. Those that stimulate insulin production, such as stress or a high consumption of carbohydrates, can lead directly to weight gain, as insulin facilitates the storage of fat.

If you have ever calorie counted, ever been under stress, ever taken antibiotics or hormones such as the pill… If you have sacrificed eating protein and fat in favour of carbohydrates… If you have eaten a lot of low-fat, low calorie, high carbohydrate foods… If you have eaten the same foods on a regular basis… If you have a weakened immune system… If you have ever eaten a less than perfect diet… You can easily have created the environment for one, or all, of Candida, Food Intolerance and Hypoglycaemia. Any one of these will lead to addict-like food cravings, further food problems and a vicious circle of problems that make you overweight and keep you overweight.

This explains why the more we count calories the more likely we are to gain weight, as we make ourselves susceptible to a multitude of problems that cause food cravings. It explains why twentieth and twenty-first century drugs and stress have contributed to the current epidemic of obesity. It explains why your cravings are so powerful that your desire to be slim alone cannot overcome them. It explains why you overeat when all you want is to be slim.

The good news is that the jigsaw can be used in our favour just as easily as it has worked against us in the past. Knowing what is happening, knowing why we have the cravings and knowing what causes what, we can use this knowledge to break the cycle and break free from overeating.

Part Four

****

The perfect diet to end overeating
The Harcombe Diet

An Introduction

For completeness, I am going to summarise The Harcombe Diet over the next three chapters. More comprehensive details, with over 100 questions and answers, can be found in my book *Stop Counting Calories & Start Losing Weight*.

The Harcombe Diet has three Phases:

Phase 1 (just five days long) is designed to do the following:

- To 'kick-start' your new way of eating with a programme that is short enough to stick to, but long enough to have a significant impact on Candida, Food Intolerance and Hypoglycaemia.
- To attack food cravings head on (by attacking the three conditions head on) when motivation and willpower are highest, at the start of a new diet.
- To achieve significant weight loss.

Phase 2 (for as long as you want to lose weight) is designed to do the following:

- To continue to win the war against Candida, Food Intolerance and Hypoglycaemia (and so to have continued impact on food cravings).
- To continue the great start made in Phase 1, but with a more varied diet, which is easier to stick to and more enjoyable.
- To change your eating habits forever. To get you eating real food and nourishing your body and to put you off processed foods and 'junk' as much as possible.

Phase 3 (for as long as you want to maintain your weight) is designed to do the following:

- To put you back in control of your eating by giving you long-term control over food cravings.
- To enable you to eat, without cravings, for life.
- To enable you to eat whatever you want, *almost* whenever you want, but with you managing the outcome.

Chapter Nine

****

Phase 1

WHAT you can eat and drink in Phase 1

Meat:

As much fresh, unprocessed, meat, as you want. This can be white meat and birds (chicken, duck, goose, guinea fowl, pheasant, quail, rabbit and turkey), or, red meat (bacon, beef, fresh ham, lamb, pork, veal and venison). Please check all ingredients, as packaged and tinned meats usually have sugars and other processed things in them. Buying from the (local) butcher, or supermarket meat counter, will be safest.

Fish:

As much fresh or tinned fish as you want – no smoked fish (because it feeds one of the conditions we're going to learn about). This can include white fish like cod, haddock, halibut, plaice, turbot and whiting. It can include oily fish like anchovies, mackerel, pilchards, salmon, tuna, and trout. It can include shellfish and seafood like clams, crab, lobster, mussels, oysters and prawns. Check that the tinned fish has no added ingredients other than oil or salt. You can cook fish in olive oil, or butter, or steam, bake or grill it.

Eggs:

As many eggs as you want (chicken, duck or any others you like). These can be cooked with butter.

Brown rice or oats:

You can have up to 50 grams (dry weight – before cooking) of whole grain brown rice per day, *or* brown rice cereal, *or* brown rice pasta, *or* porridge oats. If you are vegetarian, (or vegan), you can have up to 150 grams (dry weight) of these foods, per day, to make sure that you get enough to eat. You don't have to eat the rice or porridge, but it will give you useful energy.

Salads and Vegetables:

You can have as many salads and vegetables as you want, except mushrooms and potatoes (these are not good for two of the conditions we are going to learn about).

I've listed all that I can think of below:

- Salad stuff – alfalfa, bean sprouts, beetroot, celery, chicory, cress, cucumber, endive, all types of lettuce, radish, rocket, spring onions, watercress and a couple of fruits – olives and tomatoes.
- Vegetables – artichoke, asparagus, aubergine, bamboo shoots, broccoli, Brussels sprouts, Bok choy, cabbage, carrots, cauliflower, celeriac, chillies, courgettes, fennel, garlic, green/French beans, kale, leek, mange tout, marrow, okra, onions, parsnip, peas, peppers (any colour), pumpkin, salsify, shallots, spinach, squashes, swede, turnip, water chestnuts.
- Any herbs, spices or seasoning – basil, bay leaves, caraway, cardamom, chervil, chives, cinnamon, cloves, coriander, cumin, dill, fennel, ginger, marjoram, mint, nutmeg, oregano, paprika, parsley, pepper, rosemary, saffron, sage, salt, tarragon, thyme, turmeric.

Natural Live (Bio) Yoghurt (NLY):

We get more questions about Natural Live Yoghurt than any other food. There are only two things that you need to check:

1) Is the yoghurt live? The packet may say "live", or "bio" or "contains active cultures" or contains "lactobacillus" and so on – any or all of these are fine.

2) Is the yoghurt plain? Check that nothing else has been added – no sugar, sweetener, flavourings and so on. If the pot has nothing but yoghurt and active cultures (these are not

always listed on the label – the word live/bio is used to confirm that they are there), then it's OK to eat.

Tofu:

This is a vegetarian protein alternative, which is fine in Phase 1, provided that it doesn't contain added ingredients.

Drinks:

You can drink as much bottled water (still or sparkling) or tap water as you like during Phase 1. You can drink herbal teas, decaffeinated tea and decaffeinated coffee.

You must not drink alcohol, fruit juices, soft drinks, canned drinks (even sugar-free drinks), caffeinated products or milk. So, just to be clear, you can't have milk in tea or coffee during Phase 1.

Note:

Don't worry about mixing fats and carbs in Phase 1. Phase 1 gets the results, without adding in this Rule, which you will come across in Phase 2.

Don't eat anything that is not on the list above during Phase 1. No fruit, no wheat or grains (other than the brown rice/oat options listed), no white rice, no sugar, no cakes, no biscuits, no confectionery, no cheese, no pickled or processed foods. Don't eat anything to which you are allergic – obviously.

HOW long is Phase 1?

Phase 1 lasts for just five days. Why five days? Any food that you have eaten passes through your body in three to four days, so this gets rid of any processed foods and foods that have been causing you problems. Also, this strict part of the diet needs to be short enough for you to stick to it, but long enough to have an effect.

You can continue Phase 1 beyond five days if you have a lot of weight to lose and find it easy to stick to. This is the fastest weight loss programme I have come across, so you may be happy to put up with a restricted menu to lose weight fast.

Phase 2 adds more foods for variety and nutrients and the weight loss continues to be good, so it's up to you when you move on to the next phase.

WHEN do you eat?

All the foods allowed in Phase 1 can be eaten whenever you want. It is best to get into the habit of eating three main meals a day, with snacks in between only if you are genuinely hungry.

HOW much do you eat?

As much as you want of everything on the 'allowed' list – only the brown rice/oat options are limited. You really can have a large plate of bacon and eggs for breakfast and you can have as much meat, fish, salad and vegetables as you can eat for main meals.

If you need to snack between your three main meals then you can have cold meats, hard-boiled eggs, celery sticks, raw carrots, Natural Live Yoghurt (NLY) or a tin of tuna – whatever it takes to keep hunger away.

WHY does Phase 1 work?

Phase 1 has been scientifically designed to be the perfect diet for zapping these three conditions. Phase 1 is low carb, but not to halitosis levels. You will lose pounds, feel less bloated, and quite likely clear up a lot of other health problems along the way and all without slowing your metabolism or feeling hungry.

The small print

Just a word of caution – you may get some quite nasty withdrawal symptoms in Phase 1. You are going 'cold-turkey' on sugar and caffeine, two potentially addictive substances, and you may get some quite bad headaches if you've effectively been an addict. Taking whatever you normally take for headaches should help.

Phase 1 meal suggestions

Below are some meal options for Phase 1. Recipes for all of these menu suggestions, and lots more, can be found in *The Harcombe Diet: The Recipe Book.*

Breakfasts:

- Bacon & eggs;
- Scrambled eggs (no milk) – cooked in butter and flavoured with herbs, salt and pepper as desired;
- Plain or ham Omelette (no milk) – cooked in butter and flavoured with salt and pepper as desired;
- Natural Live Yoghurt (NLY);
- 50 grams brown rice cereal. You should be able to find this in the gluten-free section of supermarkets. (This is the 'Marmite®' of The Harcombe Diet - I love it, others hate it!);
- 50 grams porridge oats – just add boiling water and stir to the consistency you like.

Main meals (lunch/dinner):

- Any amount of meat & salad/vegetables: e.g.

    - Roast leg of lamb with rosemary & vegetables;
    - Roast chicken with garlic or lemon & vegetables;
    - Pork or lamb chops with herbs & vegetables;
    - Strips of beef or chicken & stir-fry vegetables.

- Any amount of fish/seafood & salad/vegetables: e.g.

    - Salad or salmon Niçoise (fish steak or tinned fish with hard-boiled egg(s), anchovies and green beans on a large plate of salads);
    - Mixed fish platter (chunks of cod, halibut, salmon – whatever is available) & salad/vegetables.

- Any amount of eggs & salad/vegetables: e.g.

- Omelette & salad;
- Egg and/or cold meat salad.

- Brown rice dishes: e.g.

  - Paella (seafood & chopped vegetables stir-fried with the brown rice allowance);
  - Curry & brown rice (chicken, beef, veggie curry – your usual favourite, but only using meat, fish, vegetables, herbs and spices allowed in Phase 1);
  - Stuffed tomatoes or peppers (cook the rice, add some cooked chopped vegetables and put this in a large tomato or pepper and bake in a medium oven for 20-30 minutes);
  - Home-made kebabs on brown rice (chunks of meat, fish and/or courgettes/aubergines/peppers etc);
  - Brown rice with stir-fried vegetables and/or stir-fried strips of meat.

- Vegetarian dishes: e.g.

  - Tofu & vegetables in home-made tomato sauce;
  - Tofu & stir-fry vegetables.

Starters:

- Asparagus in butter;
- A selection of soups.

Desserts:

- Just Natural Live Yoghurt for Phase 1.

Snacks – If you need to snack you can have NLY; Crudités (sticks of carrots, celery, peppers etc); hard-boiled eggs; extra meat and/or fish.

Please note that there are no chapter summaries for Chapters Nine, Ten and Eleven individually, as there is a one page summary for the diet as a whole at the end of Part Four.

Chapter Ten

****

Phase 2

WHAT you can eat and drink in Phase 2

Phase 2 has just three rules. Get to know them like the back of your hand, as this is the secret to being fit, not fat, and staying there. The three rules are:

1) Don't eat processed foods.

2) Don't eat fats and carbs at the same meal.

3) Don't eat any foods that you currently crave.

RULE NUMBER 1

Don't eat processed foods

The single simplest thing you can do to get to your ideal weight and stay there is to eat real food and absolutely nothing processed. Real food is food in the form as provided by nature. As we said in Chapter Four, oranges grow on trees, cartons of orange juice don't. Baked potatoes come out of the ground, chips don't. Cows graze in a field, Peperami® sticks don't – you get the idea.

The most commonly found processed food is sugar (sucrose) and this is particularly important to avoid, as it has no nutritional value. It gives you energy, (calories), but nothing else that you need. Avoid sugar in any form – white or brown. Anything with syrup in the title or "*ose*" at the end is usually sugar e.g. sucrose, glucose syrup, corn syrup, maltose, fructose, dextrose etc. Watch out – sugar is in cakes, biscuits, confectionery, almost every cereal, most bread, ready meals, many crisps, most desserts, many types of yoghurt and even tins of kidney beans and chickpeas.

143

Below is a list to summarise the real foods, which you should be eating and the processed foods, which you want to avoid:

DO EAT – REAL FOOD	DON'T EAT – PROCESSED FOOD
Meat: Any pure meat with no food processing e.g. pork chops, steak, lamb joints, chicken, carvery meat etc. Best sources will be the local butcher or the fresh meat counter in the grocery store. The butcher may have sausages with only meat and meat products (nothing else added) – these are fine.	Processed meats e.g. burgers, meat sticks, normal sausages etc. Tinned meats often have ingredients added – check the label. Sliced packaged meats usually have sugars, like dextrose, added.
Fish & Seafood: Any fish or seafood from the fishmongers or the fresh fish counter/aisle in the grocery store. Most tinned fish is OK – tuna, salmon, sardines – anything in just oil, brine or plain tomatoes is fine.	Processed fish – fish fingers, fish in batter, fish in breadcrumbs (contains white bread and sugar). Any microwave meals (fish or meat) invariably have sugars or other processed ingredients.
Eggs & Dairy: Any eggs. Any real milk, cheese, yoghurt, butter, cream.	Flavoured yoghurts, processed cheese sticks & slices, margarine and manufactured spreads.

DO EAT – REAL FOOD	DON'T EAT – PROCESSED FOOD
Fruit & Vegetables:	
Any whole fruits (eating the skins where edible).	Fruit juices or dried fruits e.g. raisins.
Baked potatoes with the skins on.	Chips, crisps.
Any other vegetables.	Vegetable juices, Vegetable crisps.
Grains:	
Brown rice.	White rice.
Wholemeal pasta.	White pasta.
Wholemeal flour.	White flour.
Wholemeal bread (no sugar, glucose syrup, treacle or other processed ingredients).	White bread, or any bread with sugar or sugar substances in it.
Sugar:	
Any sugar found naturally in whole food: fruit sugar in the whole fruit (fructose); milk sugar in milk (lactose).	Any sugar – white or brown; Any 'ose' added to products – e.g. maltose, dextrose, sucrose, fructose; treacle; honey etc.
Drinks:	
Water, milk, any herbal teas, Decaf tea & coffee.	Canned drinks (sugared or sweetened), fruit juice.

RULE NUMBER 2

Don't eat fat and carbs at the same meal

Do you remember from Chapter Four that food falls into two main categories, with a couple of exceptions? We have fat/proteins – foods that come from things with faces (meat, fish, eggs, dairy) and carbohydrate/proteins, which come from the ground and the trees (grains, potatoes, fruits etc). The first exceptions to note are oils, which are pure fat, with no carbohydrate or protein and sucrose (table sugar), which is pure carbohydrate, with no protein or fat.

The two really interesting food groups are carbohydrates and fats. Why are they so interesting? Because one causes the body to release a substance called insulin and the other doesn't.

Rule 2 says – eat either fat at a meal, or eat carbohydrate, but don't mix the two. The exception is that salads and vegetables have a low carbohydrate content and can, therefore, be eaten with either fat or carbohydrate meals. So your meals should be 'fat' meals (e.g. meat, fish, cheese, eggs) with salad and/or vegetables *or* 'carb' meals (e.g. brown rice, wholemeal pasta, baked potato) with salad and/or vegetables.

As a general rule, coloured and/or root vegetables, (e.g. butternut squash, carrots, parsnips etc), have a higher carb content, so go easy on these with fat meals. Potatoes (normal and sweet potatoes) should *not* be seen as vegetables – think of them as staple carbs, which form the basis of a carb meal.

The other foods to be careful of are nuts, seeds, avocados and whole milk. Nature naturally separates foods into fat/protein or carb/protein (isn't that interesting?), but these are key exceptions:
-   100 grams of peanuts, as an example, have 25 grams of carbohydrate and 51 grams of fat;
-   Sunflower seeds have 20 grams of carbohydrate and 51 grams of fat; and
-   Avocado has 9 grams of carbohydrate and 15 grams of fat. These are real and nutritious foods, but not great for weight loss.

Finally, milk and yoghurt are the interesting animal foods. Meat and fish are totally carb free. Eggs, cheese and cream are virtually carb free, but milk and yoghurt, both low-fat and real, have approximately five grams of carbohydrate per 100 grams. This is still very low in carbohydrate, but go easy on the lattés and NLY – especially between meals.

On the following page there is a useful list to show which foods can be eaten as a fat meal and which can be eaten as a carb meal and which can be eaten with either. If you're allergic to anything in here, e.g. fish, then obviously don't eat it.

FAT MEALS	CARB MEALS
Any unprocessed meat –bacon, beef, chicken, duck, goose, guinea fowl, ham, lamb, pheasant, pork, quail, rabbit, turkey, veal, venison	All **Fruit**
	Whole grains – brown rice, brown pasta, brown rice pasta, couscous, 100% wholemeal bread, quinoa, millet etc.
Any unprocessed fish – cod, haddock, halibut, mackerel, plaice, pilchards, salmon, seafood, trout, tuna, whiting etc. Includes tinned fish in only oil, salt and/or water	**Wholemeal cereal** – porridge oats, Brown rice cereal, Shredded Wheat®, other sugar-free cereal
Eggs – Chicken, duck etc.	**Beans & Pulses** – lentils, broad beans, kidney beans, chickpeas etc.
Dairy Products – Cheese, milk, butter, cream, yoghurt (ideally Natural Live Yoghurt)	Baked **Potatoes** in their skins

EAT WITH EITHER A FAT OR A CARB MEAL

Salads – alfalfa, bean sprouts, beetroot, celery, chicory, cress, cucumber, endive, all types of lettuce, radish, rocket, spring onions etc.

Vegetables – artichoke, asparagus, aubergine, bamboo shoots, broccoli, Brussels sprouts, cabbage, carrot, cauliflower, celeriac, chillies, courgettes, garlic, green beans, kale, leek, mange tout, marrow, okra, onions, parsnip, peas, peppers (any colour), pumpkin, salsify, shallots, spinach, squashes, swede, turnip, water chestnuts etc.

Tofu/Quorn – Vegetarian protein alternatives

Certain **Fruits** – olives, tomatoes & berries

Low-fat dairy products – milk, cottage cheese & yoghurt

Herbs, Spices & Seasoning – basil, chives, coriander, cumin, dill, fennel, mint, oregano, paprika, parsley, pepper, rosemary, sage, salt, thyme etc. Olive oil for cooking.

How to use this list:

1) You can eat anything on the fat list with anything on the 'eat with either' list. You can eat anything on the carb list with anything on the 'eat with either' list.

2) You should *not* eat anything on the fat and carb lists at the same meal.

3) Generally, when fat is removed from a product something else needs to be put back in to replace it. The exception to this is with animal fat products, where fat can be removed and nothing needs to be put back in its place. So, where there are low-fat alternatives to standard products like milk and yoghurt, these can be eaten with carb meals. This lets us have skimmed milk with cereals and low-fat cottage cheese with baked potatoes, for example.

4) The fruits on the 'eat with either' list, (olives, tomatoes and berries), have a carb content more like vegetables, than fruit and so they can be eaten with either fat meals or carb meals. (Don't eat olives by the bucket load, with carb meals, however, as olives also have a reasonable fat content). These fruits give the diet some great menu options, as it means you can have berries and low-fat yoghurt after a carb meal. It also means that you can have tomato pasta sauces, as well as using tomatoes and olives in meat and fish dishes.

5) Try to leave three to four hours between a fat meal and a carb meal, because this is the time that food normally takes to be digested. You should achieve this naturally by having three meals a day. If you are eating snacks (not ideal), have carb snacks between carb meals and fat snacks between fat meals (the menu plan at the back gives you an illustration).

RULE NUMBER 3

Don't eat foods that you currently crave

The clue to which condition (or all three) that you have is what you crave...

If you have **Candida** (classic symptoms are dandruff, athlete's foot and a white coating in your mouth when you wake up), you are likely to crave bread, pizza, beer, cereal, biscuits, sweets, pickled foods and blue cheese. You will need to avoid these and limit all carbs, even fruit, in Phase 2.

If you have **Food Intolerance**, you will crave the thing(s) to which you are intolerant. The most common food intolerances are the things that we eat every day – wheat, milk and sugar being the main culprits. Be honest, whichever food(s) you really feel you couldn't live without are the ones you need to give up. You won't have to give them up forever, but just until you've lost weight and got your immune system back in good shape. Then you'll be able to re-introduce them (you just won't be able to have too much of them and too often).

Classic symptoms of **Hypoglycaemia** are: waking at 4am hungry and possibly with night sweats; an 11am and 4pm 'dip' during the day, where you feel irritable, hungry and unable to make a decision; and general cravings for sweets and sweet foods. These foods then give you an instant sugar rush, followed by an energy dip and cravings for more sweet foods. If you have Hypoglycaemia, limit all carbs in Phase 2 and have as many fat meals as possible. Have no more than one to two pieces of fruit per day during Phase 2 and go for lower sugar fruits like apples, pears, citrus fruits and berries. Avoid tropical fruits, like bananas, melons and so on.

If you have more than one condition, you will need to follow the advice for all the conditions that affect you. This will restrict the foods that you can eat, but this is only until your immune system recovers and your body can tolerate your problem foods again. You are not giving up these foods forever.

HOW long is Phase 2?

Follow Phase 2 for as long as you want to lose weight. If you have a stone (14 pounds) or less to lose then you could easily lose five to seven pounds in Phase 1 and you may only need to follow Phase 2 for a couple more weeks. If you have a lot of weight to lose then you can be free from hunger and food cravings throughout Phase 2 and you will lose weight while eating healthy, natural foods, which your body will thank you for.

WHEN do you eat?

Eat whenever you want, in Phase 2, but try to get into the habit of eating three substantial meals a day and only snacking in between if you are genuinely hungry.

Now that you know that insulin is the fattening hormone, you know that the fewer times you raise your blood glucose level during the day, the better. If you snack on low-fat/high carb foods, you are causing your body to release insulin on a more regular basis and this won't help you to lose weight.

Just as insulin facilitates fat storage, so it prevents fat burning. Eating a carbohydrate 'injects' glucose and insulin into the blood stream and this has been shown to diminish the level of fatty acids almost immediately. Until the carb, glucose and insulin arrived, the fatty acids were being used for fuel. You want to optimise the hours during which your body is using fat for fuel and not glucose – another reason not to snack.

HOW much do you eat?

Eat what you need. However, just because quantities are unlimited doesn't mean that you're training for an eating contest. Don't go hungry, but don't go mad either. One of the many reasons that this diet works so well is that you will find it almost impossible to overeat. The body has a natural appetite mechanism when given only real food.

WHY does Phase 2 work?

The rationale behind Phase 2 is really simple and powerful:

Rule 1 – Don't eat processed foods

This is because when you eat processed foods your body is highly likely to release too much insulin (e.g. if you drink orange juice, your body thinks you have eaten several oranges and pumps out enough insulin to mop up lots of oranges). We must stop this happening for two key reasons:

1) As insulin is the fattening hormone we want our bodies to release the right amount of insulin to mop up the food we have actually eaten, not too much, or else the extra is stored as fat. If we eat the whole orange or whole grains, i.e. the whole food every time, our bodies should release the right amount of insulin.

2) If we end up with too much insulin, after eating something, our blood glucose level will be low, which will make us crave food to get our blood glucose level back to normal. So, we will have cravings for food – especially processed foods – which is what has made us eat junk and put on weight in the first place.

Processed foods are 'empty calories'. They give us calories, i.e. energy/fuel, but they don't give us as many vitamins and minerals (nutrients) as we could get from eating the same number of calories from real food. If we don't get the nutrients we need, we will crave foods to find other ways of getting these nutrients. If we eat a varied diet of real food – meat, fish, eggs, dairy products, vegetables, salad and fruit – we will be more likely to get the nutrients we need and our body won't need to crave things. If we eat microwave meals, cakes and biscuits and so on, we are going to crave more food to get the nutrients.

Rule 2 – Don't eat fats and carbohydrates at the same meal

The easiest substance for the body to get energy from is carbohydrate. So, if your body spots that you've eaten a carb it says "Thank you very much – I'll use that for my immediate energy needs and I'll store any fat with it for later on". The double whammy is that the body needs insulin to store fat, and it is only carbohydrates that cause insulin to be released. So, your body can only store that fat, for later on, when you have eaten a carbohydrate.

As an example, if you eat a bacon butty the body will take the bread and tomato sauce carbs for immediate energy and store the bacon and butter for later on. *And* the body is only able to store the fat because insulin has been released and this only happened because of the bread and tomato sauce. The 'great' British diet is based on mixing fats and carbs: Cheddar ploughman's; fish and chips; roast beef and Yorkshire pudding – no wonder we're overweight.

If you eat carbohydrate, and no fat, the body uses the carbs for energy and there is no fat to store. If you eat fat, and no carbohydrate, your body has to use the fat for energy and it has to work a bit harder to do this (which is good news for you, because it naturally uses up more energy). As we don't want to facilitate fat storage, we don't want to eat these two food groups at the same time.

Rule 3 – **Don't eat foods that you currently crave**

You crave the foods that feed any of the three conditions, from which you may be suffering, because Candida, Food Intolerance and Hypoglycaemia all lead to unbelievable food cravings. To lose weight comfortably, you have to stop the cravings. To stop the cravings you have to get these three conditions back under control.

Phase 2 meal suggestions

Below are some meal options for Phase 2. Recipes for all of these menu suggestions, and lots more, can be found in *The Harcombe Diet: The Recipe Book*.

You can have a fat meal or a carb meal whenever you like. The more fat meals you have, the quicker you will lose weight (carbs and insulin really are the secret to weight loss). However, do balance this with the nutrients and menu variety that come with good carbs and enjoy carb meals as part of Phase 2.

With all of the following, don't forget to add in Rule 3 and avoid the food(s) that you crave... So, limit fruit to one to two pieces a day for Candida and Hypoglycaemia and have rice pasta, instead of wheat pasta, and no bread, if you have wheat intolerance.

Breakfasts – fat meals

- Bacon & eggs (no ketchup or brown sauce);
- Kippers/smoked haddock;
- Scrambled eggs;
- Plain, ham or cheese omelette;
- Natural Live Yoghurt (NLY);
- Cooking options for fat breakfasts include grilling, poaching, steaming, baking or frying in butter or vegetable oil.

Breakfasts – carb meals

- Fruit platter (optional low-fat NLY);
- Shredded Wheat® & skimmed milk (with a sliced banana – optional);
- Brown rice cereal (with skimmed milk or great on its own, as it stays crunchy);
- 100% porridge oats with water, or skimmed milk;
- Sugar-free muesli with water, or skimmed milk;
- Wholemeal bread & marmite.

Main meals – starters – fat meals

- Prawn cocktail;
- Tomatoes & mozzarella;
- Asparagus in butter;
- Salmon & cream cheese;
- A selection of soups.

154

Main meals – starters – carb meals

- Char grilled vegetables with olive oil or balsamic;
- Vegetable kebabs;
- Melon selection;
- Fruit salad;
- A selection of soups.

Main meals – main courses – fat meals

- Any amount of meat & salad/vegetables: e.g.

    - Roast leg of lamb with rosemary & vegetables;
    - Roast chicken with garlic or lemon & vegetables;
    - Pork or lamb chops with herbs & vegetables;
    - Strips of beef or chicken & stir-fry vegetables.
    - Ham, egg, cold meat salad (Chef's salad);

- Any amount of fish/seafood & salad/vegetables: e.g.

    - Tuna or salmon Niçoise (fish steak or tinned fish with hard-boiled egg(s), anchovies & green beans on a large plate of salads);
    - Mixed fish platter (chunks of cod, halibut, salmon – whatever is available) & salad/vegetables.

- Any amount of eggs/cheese & salad/vegetables: e.g.

    - Omelette (with or without cheese) & salad;
    - Four cheese salad;
    - Cauliflower cheese and/or cheesy leeks;
    - Egg & asparagus bake;
    - Egg and/or cold meat salad.

- Vegetarian dishes: e.g.

    - Tofu & vegetables in home-made tomato sauce;
    - Quorn & vegetables in home-made tomato sauce;
    - Tofu or Quorn & stir-fry vegetables.

155

Main meals – main courses – carb meals

- Brown rice & stir-fry vegetables;
- Quinoa with stir-fry vegetables;
- Wholemeal pasta & tomato sauce;
- Wholemeal spaghetti & tomato sauce;
- Vegetarian chilli & brown rice;
- Couscous & char grilled vegetables;
- Vegetarian curry & brown rice;
- Baked potato & salad and/or very low-fat cottage cheese and/or ratatouille;
- Roasted vegetables with pine nuts & Parmesan cheese;
- Stuffed tomatoes and/or stuffed peppers.

Main meals – desserts – fat meals

- Strawberries (or any berries) & yoghurt or cream;
- Sugar-free ice cream;
- Natural Live Yoghurt;
- Greek Yoghurt (can be full fat with a fat meal);
- Cheese selection (no crackers or grapes).

Main meals – desserts – carb meals

- Any berries with very low-fat yoghurt (e.g. strawberries, raspberries, blackberries etc).

A note here on fruit: fruit salad is the obvious carb dessert, but don't go for this. Eat fruit alone or before any other food. Fruit digests in less than half an hour. Some foods take about four hours. If you eat fruit after steak, for example, the fruit gets stuck behind the meat in the digestive tract and your stomach will bloat. The only exception to this is berries – you can eat strawberries, raspberries etc at the end of a meal, as relative to other fruits, they are very high in water content, high in dietary fibre and low in sugar. Strawberries for example are 92% water vs. a banana at 74%. Blackberries have five times the dietary fibre of an apple (per 100 grams) and dietary fibre passes through the stomach undigested and more slowly. Raspberries have half the sugar content of apples.

Snacks – fat options

- Cheese;
- Hard-boiled eggs;
- Natural Live Yoghurt;
- Cold cuts of meat.

Snacks – either

- Crudités (sticks of carrots, celery, peppers etc).

Snacks – carb options

- Sugar-free cereal bars – ideally wheat-free also. Health food shops have a reasonable selection;
- Sugar-free oat biscuits (ingredients of oats, oil & salt only);
- Fruit (ideally lower sugar fruits like apples, pears, citrus fruits and berries);
- Rice cakes (high Glycaemic Index, so avoid these if you are very carb sensitive).

Easy lunches for work – fat meals

- Tinned tuna/salmon with salad in a lunch box;
- Cold meat (chicken/turkey/beef/ham) with salad;
- Any fat leftovers from dinner the night before;
- Frittata – cold omelette.

Easy lunches for work – carb meals

- Brown bread sandwich with anything low-fat e.g. salad, hummus, cottage cheese;
- The 'national dish' of Israel: wholemeal pita bread stuffed with falafel and salad;
- Brown rice salad – cold brown rice with chopped salad ingredients;

- Any carb leftovers from dinner the night before;
- Baked potato & salad and/or low-fat cottage cheese;
- Fruit platter.

A note here on wheat intolerance: you may well find wholemeal pita bread OK, even if normal bread causes bloating and other problems.

Chapter Eleven

****

Phase 3

This chapter is the secret of how to have your cake and eat it. This is about eating as much as you can get away with, without putting on weight. It will take a bit of trial and error, but, once you've got it, you'll never look back.

Move onto Phase 3 when you are at what we call your 'natural weight'. This is the weight that you can maintain easily – going above it takes some overeating and going below it only happens when you are ill or under stress. Some men call this their 'fighting weight' – it's what you feel good at, but can also stay at without too much effort.

WHAT can you eat and drink/not eat or drink?

The three rules from Phase 2 should still form the basis of your eating in Phase 3. These really are your top tips for lifelong healthy eating.

The difference with Phase 3 is that you can also eat what you want *almost* when you want. This is called 'cheating'. The key thing is to make sure that you don't start putting weight back on and here is how you do this:

1) Don't 'cheat' too much;

2) Don't 'cheat' too often;

3) Be alert and stay in control.

Number 1 says don't 'cheat' too much – eat a confectionery bar if you want one, but don't eat ten. Eat a dessert if you want one, but don't eat the bread sticks while you're waiting for your starter. Rule Number 1 is, therefore, about the *quantity* of the processed foods that you eat.

Number 2 says don't 'cheat' too often. Have a dessert for a special occasion, but just not every day. Eat that confectionery bar if you want to, but not every day. Number 2 is, therefore, about the *frequency* with which you eat processed foods. Try to stick to the rules in Phase 2 as often as possible and then only cheat when you really fancy something.

Number 3, is about you having the knowledge and the skills to control your cravings and, therefore, to control your eating and your weight. Get to know what works for you. You may get it wrong the first time and you may find that cravings return. Don't panic. Go back to Phase 2 for however long it takes to get back in control.

To learn from the experience ask yourself some questions – Were you cheating too much (quantity)? Were you cheating too often (frequency)? You were probably more than half aware that you were starting to become quite attached to a particular food or foods and, therefore, you should have cut back earlier as this was the first sign of cravings. Be really honest with yourself next time and as soon as you think you *need* something rather than *want* something, avoid that food totally, for at least five days.

Top tips for becoming a master of cheating

The basics are all you need – don't cheat too much, don't cheat too often and be alert and stay in control. However, if you want to become a gold medallist at cheating, here are the top tips...

Tip 1 – Cheat all at once

If you want a pizza, eat a pizza, but don't keep eating one or two slices throughout the day. Remember, you are trying to minimise the number of times your pancreas releases insulin.

Tip 2 – Eat as few ingredients as possible

The fewer processed ingredients you can attack your body with the better. If you have a packet of crisps, pick the one that has just potatoes and vegetable oil (you don't even need salt).

There are some packets of crisps that have more than 100 ingredients in them – steer well clear of these.

If you want ice cream then a quality vanilla ice cream need only contain (in order) fresh cream, skimmed milk, sugar, egg yolk and natural vanilla flavouring. Such simple and largely real ingredients tastes as good as ice cream can get. Don't pick the carton with more ingredients than you can recognise let alone remember.

Tip 3 – Have a strategy for getting your blood glucose level back to normal

If you eat a processed food, your body will almost certainly release too much insulin and this will make your blood glucose level fall lower than before you ate the substance. Your body will then demand food to get your blood glucose level back to normal. This is the time when you are most at risk of craving another processed food. So, anticipate that this will happen and have something healthy to hand when you feel your blood glucose level drop. This can be a piece of fruit or an oat biscuit – any whole food that will get your blood glucose level back to normal naturally.

Tip 4 – Don't eat your normal meal AND cheat

If you are going to have a bag of kettle chips for lunch then make that your lunch. Don't have your steak and salad as well, as your body will just store the fat in the steak when you eat the kettle chip carbs.

Tip 5 – Don't waste cheating

If you are going out for dinner don't start on the nuts and bread sticks before dinner – you know you'll eat them all as soon as you start, so don't even have one. Save your cheating for the real food and enjoy something really special from the menu instead.

Tip 6 – Don't forget that insulin is the fattening hormone

Carbohydrates stimulate the production of insulin, the fattening hormone, but so do caffeine and sweeteners. You may like to return to full caffeine coffee and cola in Phase 3, but this must be counted as cheating. If this is really how you want to use your cheating then do so. Cheating connoisseurs never forget that the key to cheating is to minimise the production of insulin.

Tip 7 – Have exactly what you want

If you want a pint of Guinness, don't settle for a low-carb beer instead. You'll only have the low-carb beer and then still want the Guinness, so just have it.

Tip 8 – Just because you can cheat doesn't mean you have to

This diet lets you eat every real food on the planet – meat, fish, eggs, dairy products, fruits, salads, vegetables, whole grains. You will not miss out on anything by not eating processed foods so, if you don't have any urge to 'cheat', then don't.

The Harcombe Diet – A Summary

Phase 1 – 5 days

- **Do eat** meat, fish, eggs, (tofu – if you are tolerant to soy products), Natural Live Yoghurt, any salads, any vegetables (except potatoes or mushrooms), some brown rice, herbs and spices, olive oil and butter.

- **Do drink** still or sparkling water, herbal teas, decaffeinated tea or coffee.

- **Don't eat** anything that is not on the list above. No fruit, no wheat or grains (other than brown rice) no white rice, no sugar, no cakes, no biscuits, no confectionery, no cheese, no pickled or processed foods.

- **Don't drink** alcohol, fruit juices, soft drinks, low calorie soft drinks, caffeinated products or milk.

Phase 2 – while you need to lose weight

- **Rule 1** – Don't eat processed foods.

- **Rule 2** – Don't eat fats and carbohydrates at the same meal.

- **Rule 3** – Don't eat foods that cause *your* cravings.

Phase 3 – Life long weight maintenance

- Don't cheat too much.

- Don't cheat too often.

- Be alert and stay in control.

Part Five

****

The mindset to end overeating

Chapter Twelve

The six basic emotions & overeating

Emotional reasons for eating and overeating

Having explored the physical reasons for overeating, let us now turn to the emotional reasons. As Chapter One shared, I used to work as a Human Resources Director and one of the best training courses I have ever attended was with the Australian founders of the Restorative Justice process. Restorative Justice is also known as 'conflict resolution conferencing' and the idea is that people in conflict are brought together to resolve their differences by talking. It works for two reasons:

1) The average human being would rather be in harmony with others than in conflict.

2) The power of the group (mob mentality) will work to help individuals in conflict tend towards harmony.

I mention this because one of the most fascinating parts of the course was about our six basic emotions. We learned on the course how to recognise these emotions, through words and body language, so that we could harness them to achieve group harmony.

We have six basic emotions that we express as human beings. The words in the English language that best describe them are:

- Interest
- Fear
- Surprise
- Distress
- Anger
- Enjoyment

We eat for many reasons and many of these reasons are related to our emotions. The key reason for eating should be to feed our body, to nourish it by giving it the vitamins and minerals that it needs. Our ancestors did tend to eat for this reason and for them food was about survival. They needed enough food to keep warm and to keep starvation and illness away. We seem to eat now for almost any reason other than that we are hungry or require vitamins and minerals. We tend to eat for emotional reasons so let us look at these six basic emotions...

Interest – We do eat out of curiosity. We eat because we want to know what something tastes like. If we have eaten chocolate cake before, we want to see what that particular chocolate cake tastes like. Even if we can pretty much guarantee what something will taste like, we still seem to want to eat that substance to see what it will taste like right now in this moment.

Fear – On the course, real fear was one of the most important emotions that could be observed on people's faces, as conflict resolution conferencing could be highly emotional. Human beings tend not to eat when facing genuine fear. The last thing on a hijack victim's mind is food. When experiencing a nasty road rage attack, people are not thinking about food. We do tend to eat, however, when faced with mild and perhaps inappropriate fear. Have you ever been to a supermarket the day before a public holiday? Do we stockpile or do we stockpile?! It is as if we fear running out of food. I have never known anyone die of starvation over Thanksgiving, Yom Kippur, Ramadan, Christmas or any other celebratory festival. Yet we shop and eat as if this is bound to happen.

This 'fear' of going without food is by no means limited to the handful of days each year that the shops are closed. We fear going without food for even a few hours. How many people eat in the airport terminal because they don't know when their next meal is due? How many people eat the aeroplane food for exactly the same reason – we don't know when we will land, when we will get to our destination, when the next meal will be. Only diabetics might need food with this kind of certainly and regularity. The rest of us are eating it a) because it is there and b) because of the bizarre sense of fear of when we will next come across food. (My suggestion for not knowing when the next meal is due is to carry a small bar of high cocoa content chocolate with you when travelling and then you will always know that you can stave off genuine hunger if you need to).

Surprise – In conflict conferencing, surprise is a fascinating emotion as this is how the real breakthroughs are made. When dawning realisations occur to all parties as to why other people did what they did, the most difficult relationships can turn full circle. In our generally less serious day to day world, surprise is a rare emotion. Think about the last time something really surprised you. When did you last have that wonderful expression on your face that surprise elicits?

With eating it is almost certainly the *lack* of surprise in our daily lives that makes us eat, rather than surprise itself. Lack of surprise is of course boredom. How often do you eat because you are bored? You're in a dull meeting and the lunch sandwiches arrive and you see it as the answer to your prayers. At least now you have something fun to do. You are waiting in a queue, in traffic, to collect the children, for someone to arrive and I bet you think of food way more than even you normally would. You are bored. You are lacking surprise in your life.

Do you remember what your parents said when you told them that you were bored? "Only boring people get bored." Ouch – how much did that one hurt? There's usually more than a grain of truth in things that hurt. We may express boredom with food, but it may well go deeper.

I sometimes hear people saying I'm bored with the food I can eat on The Harcombe Diet and three things spring to mind:

1) I wonder if what they really mean is they have little interest in meat/fish/eggs/veg because what they really fancy is chocolate, croissants, cereal and the things that they used to

eat. Having little interest in foods that are good for you is more of an indication of feeling addicted to other foods, than it is in really thinking that you don't want to eat the most nutritious foods on the planet. It wouldn't make sense for you *not* to be interested in the healthiest foods.

2) When you say that you're bored, are you bored with food or bored with life? Food is one of our most routine things. We tend to get into patterns with breakfast, lunch, dinners, where we eat, what we eat, the times we eat and so on. If the rest of our life is interesting and varied, food routine can be quite reassuring and comforting. If the rest of our life is also routine and 'boring', we genuinely will miss the variety and stimulus of bingeing/starving/doing different diets/trying different foods and so on.

Take a really honest look at your life at the moment. Is it too mundane? Can you predict how the next week, fortnight, month is going to pan out? Do you have little to look forward to? Do you have nothing that will really surprise or excite you? If this is the case, you will inevitably be driven towards 'comfort eating', as your life lacks the surprise and excitement that we need as human beings and you are using food as a way to fill this void.

3) Food has assumed an unnatural importance in our previous lives – it is natural to think that something is missing when we don't spend all of our time eating or trying not to eat or trying different diets. Trying different diets in itself was not boring. We might have been trying different diets all the time or reading different diet books. We now have the answer – eat real food. No more diet books or strange diets needed. The only debate now is – which real food might I also avoid for other reasons? Nuts? Dairy? Fruit?

Tips for boredom:

-   What are you really bored with? There are still cultures on the planet today living on buffalo meat and milk and virtually nothing else. Eskimos are living on vegetation and animals that they can get from the sea. We can't really be bored with steak, roast lamb, pork chops, omelettes, hundreds of different fish dishes and vegetable accompaniments. Many of us will also be able to enjoy grains and dairy foods, berries & baked potatoes. Is it food that you are bored with or life generally? Do you feel stuck in a rut and food was the one escape that you relished? Feeling bored could be a wonderful kick start to re-evaluate things and start doing more of things that you want to do. (I can sympathise as a former veggie with this one. I got to my natural weight and enjoyed great variety as a veggie, but I never had to go super low carb. I have always been OK with rice, rice pasta, porridge, dairy foods and dark chocolate for example. If you are very carb sensitive and vegetarian, your staples will be very limited. I would be less worried about the boredom and more worried that you would develop new Food Intolerances by eating the same things day after day).

- Know your personality type – if you're someone who likes routine, the same foods eaten regularly shouldn't bother you. If you need more variety – develop an interest in cooking and recipes and make the things that you should be eating as interesting as possible.
- Bear in mind that an obsession with food and dieting is a full time job. You need to work out what you're going to do when you no longer have an eating problem. You will have so much time freed up and many of us need to work out what to do with all this spare time.

Distress – Now we get into a really interesting emotion when it comes to food. Extreme distress is likely to stop people eating. When people suffer bereavement, or the end of a special relationship, they suffer extreme distress and often eat considerably less than they would normally. People have been known to lose pounds after the loss of a family member or during divorce. Genuine and extreme distress, like genuine and extreme fear, generally takes away our emotional need for food. Again, as with fear, it is the milder and more regular distress that we suffer day to day that drives us to eat for

170

emotional reasons. Another word for distress is sadness. When we are generally sad, as opposed to the huge trauma of loss, we tend to eat for emotional reasons. We eat to cheer ourselves up. We didn't get the job we wanted, the person we fancy doesn't fancy us, we are feeling low because the dark nights are drawing in, we are just having one of those blue periods in life – this is when we reach for food as a comfort. We literally look to food to cheer us up. The real sadness is that it doesn't work. If food did cheer us up, the world would be a much happier place than it is now.

When we eat, we don't just deal with sadness. A lot of other emotions come into play. We feel the initial high of the food getting into our bodies (or literally the blood glucose level rising in our bodies, as we now understand) but the more we eat the guiltier we feel. The angrier we feel at ourselves, the more disappointed and so on. We feel all kinds of emotions but we rarely feel cheered up, which was the reason for eating in the first place.

Anger – is a fascinating emotion. Entire books have been written about anger and food. There is actually a physical reason why we eat when we are angry. Anger triggers the 'fright, flight, fight' mechanism in our bodies. The anger physically causes adrenalin to be released into the blood, because the body is getting ready to deal with the crisis and to help us 'fight' or 'flight' (run away). The problem is, when we are sitting in our cars and we experience road rage (either ourselves or against us), the fright, flight, fight mechanism works beautifully. The body gets itself ready for the fight or for running away, and yet nothing happens. We rarely confront the other driver, so all the adrenalin that was there ready for the battle has nowhere to go. It sits within us instead and we just have to live with the rage. Physically and emotionally we are now heading towards a huge urge to eat. Physically our blood glucose level is just about to drop, because the adrenalin rushing around has not been dealt with. Emotionally we have all this rage that has not been dealt with and it turns inwards instead. We feel so angry and yet we have not had a chance to

171

get even. We get even with a box of chocolates or a packet of biscuits instead.

Two inspirational trainers, with whom I had the great pleasure of working, gave me an insight into anger that has had a profound effect on my thinking. Kevin Downey and Brad Waldron, told me that "Anger is a pill that you swallow hoping to make someone else ill." We can lie there at three o'clock in the morning feeling rage towards another person and yet they have absolutely no idea that we are doing this. We are the ones feeling the rage, hoping that they will feel the pain. They don't, we do.

Think about all the times that you eat out of anger or frustration and start being alert to your emotional reasons for eating. Your partner didn't do what you wanted them to do so you feel angry and turn to food. The children are driving you mad so you eat. Your boss or work colleagues are making you angry so you seek solace in food. Your family are making unreasonable demands of you and not considering your needs. Who in fact is suffering for all the anger you are feeling? Not the other people that is for sure. Don't swallow this anger pill, and all the emotional turmoil that goes with it, because it doesn't have the desired effect on the person or situation you are angry with. It can, however, have a profound and damaging effect on you.

Enjoyment – is the final basic emotion that we are exploring in relation to food. This has quite obvious connections with why we eat. We eat when we are sad and we eat when we are happy. Human beings don't seem to need an excuse to eat. Often when we are ecstatically happy we don't eat. When we fall in love, or when our wedding day is approaching, or when we are about to go on a trip of a lifetime, we often feel so happy that we don't eat and people can lose pounds in the early days of a new relationship. However, as we saw with fear and distress, it is only in the extreme of an emotion that we tend *not* to eat. When we feel moderately happy or content we can turn to food to try to give us even more enjoyment. Once the new relationship has gone past the really exciting first few days or weeks, quite often people put back on the weight that they lost and more. The happy couple have breakfast in bed together, they go out for dinner, they have picnics in the park, they 'spoil' each other with chocolates and other edible gifts and the weight soon goes back on.

We eat when we feel contentment, therefore, and we eat because we think it will give us enjoyment. We eat emotionally for the pleasure we think that food will give us. However, the enjoyment is very short lived. As the saying goes – a minute in the mouth and a lifetime on the hips. We get very brief enjoyment from eating processed carbohydrates in particular as they are so easy to swallow. Nature's own food delights, such as mangos or pineapples, take longer to eat and chew and can, therefore, be even more enjoyable.

We also eat because we think it will make enjoyable experiences even more so. We go to the cinema and we eat ice cream, M&M's® and popcorn and wash it down with additive filled fizzy drinks. Does this really make the movie more enjoyable? Does it make us feel good inside? There are so many emotional reasons behind why we eat that are related to enjoyment. We eat because we are enjoying something or because we think it will make us enjoy that something more.

A final point to make in relation to eating for enjoyment is that, when you are addicted to a particular food, you move quickly from eating that food for enjoyment, to eating it to avoid the opposite of enjoyment, which is what happens when you don't have it. This means that you will no longer feel enjoyment when you eat a food to which you are addicted. However, you will feel bad if you don't eat it because you will have withdrawal symptoms and so you mistakenly think you will feel enjoyment if you do have it. Only when you are no longer addicted to food can you really savour tastes and genuinely enjoy food. Until then, the food is controlling you, rather than the other way round.

We tend to eat, therefore, when we are not experiencing the real extremes of our basic emotions but when we are in that middle band of 'normal' life. However, this means that for the vast majority of our lives, during this normal range, we have emotional drivers to make us eat. We don't seem to need an excuse to eat and yet there are many – boredom, road rage, travel, public holidays and new relationships – anything and everything that happens to us in life seems to have an emotional connection to food. Why is this?

Quick summary of Chapter Twelve

- There are six basic human emotions. The words that best describe these are: interest; fear; surprise; distress; anger and enjoyment.

- We tend *not* to eat when faced with the extremes of these basic emotions – at our most scared, distressed or happy.

- It is the milder levels of these emotions that can stimulate overeating – curiosity, contentment and so on.

Chapter Thirteen

****

The impact of childhood

There is a saying that goes something like "Show me the child of seven and I will show you the adult." This states that the child of seven has experienced the vast majority of the development in life that they will go through and, therefore, their preferences, personality traits and behaviour are all determined at this early age. Some people now suggest that seven is late and that the final personality is formed in most people as early as the age of three or four. So, for any of you with children older than seven, the argument says that your work is over – there is not much that you can do now to change how your child is going to be in later life. What a thought!

The four pillars of childhood

The four pillars of childhood are the four necessary conditions for a person's esteem to develop positively in these key formative years.

I learned about these while studying for a Diploma in Clinical Weight Management and these were core to the part of the syllabus on eating disorders. I have added a Pillar 0 – a precursor to the others being possible – and this is that our own parents and primary carers had high self-esteem and good mental health, during our formative years. It is very difficult for an adult to give a child the healthy nurturing that it needs, if the adult's own childhood was not a nurturing experience. Some particularly unaware adults can even 'take out' their deficiencies on children in a particularly destructive way. Pillar 0 is quite a hurdle to set at the outset, and then four more are needed. It is little wonder that one in four people in the UK will experience mental health problems in the course of any year (The Mental Health Foundation).

Here are the four pillars, which infants need in their formative years:

1) Unconditional love and positive reinforcement from our parents and/or primary carers.

The child has to know that s/he is completely loved and valued, without conditions; otherwise a sense of feeling worthless can so easily develop. Conditional love occurs when a parent places a condition on their love for the child e.g. "I don't love you when you're naughty" (this implies that the child is only loved when they are 'good', whatever good means). "Only children who eat their greens are allowed to have ice cream." This directly links food into emotional situations, at a formative age and it sets conditions such as – I will only do nice things for you (give you ice cream) if you do what I want (eat your greens). Such conditions are confusing for a child and quite possibly destructive.

2) Discipline – All children need accompanying boundaries to go with this unconditional love.

A dog cannot be content without knowing its place in 'the pack', as, in the absence of direction, it thinks that it is the master and stresses about the responsibility that this brings. Children, similarly, needs to know what they can and can't do, or they get overloaded with decision making. They will push the boundaries – this is part of growing up – but the boundaries need to be there and they need to be reasonable and consistent. No boundaries can be as stressful as too many boundaries (the dog example); unreasonable boundaries are harmful (e.g. children have to be out of sight when adults are around) and inconsistent boundaries literally mess with the minds of young children, as they are trying to get some sense of order in the world around them. A strict bed time of 5pm one night, then 9pm another, then 7pm another – without any reasonable reason for this – is destructive discipline.

3) Encouragement and respect from our parents and/or primary carers, during the formative years (and beyond) for our own personal development.

Acknowledgement that we are important, our opinions count, adults not being dismissive and so on. Sports coaches learn that you should deliver at least six or seven positive messages for every one corrective message. Even where the correction is helpful, e.g. "you need to commit earlier to the tackle", the sports person needs half a dozen other "well done's", "Great job" to get the right balance of encouragement. We almost can't tell children too often how wonderful they are, how well they have just done, and so on, to cement this pillar of esteem.

4) Self Control – By this we mean "control of the self", the sense of control for oneself – feeling safe and having one's own space.

If any seriously negative conditions are present for the infant, like abuse, hunger, cold or serious neglect, for example, this will violate the heart of any sense of having control of their self. Abuse of a young child can take many forms and it is well-documented that possibly the worst kind of abuse is neglect and ignoring the child. This goes to the core of a person not being 'validated' and therefore literally not feeling 'valid' or entitled to be part of the world.

In order, a child would much prefer 1) positive attention and good parenting; 2) negative attention and bad parenting (at least they have some attention) and the worst case scenario is 3) no attention. I am always fascinated by the parallels with animals and children – particularly dogs, a man's best friend. A dog too would rather be beaten by its master (attention) than abandoned or ignored. Being ignored by the master is the dog's worst nightmare.

Control of the self goes beyond the need to feel safe. It is vitally important to feel that we have control over our lives to the right extent at the right age. An appropriate element of control must be given over to a child at the right age all the time. If your parents rarely let you decide basic things: what to wear; what to eat; when to eat; when to sleep; when to wake up; who to play with, and so on – and particularly where this showed little change as you got older, you did not have adequate control of the self.

This is one of the major precursors of anorexia. As anorexia is primarily about control – the teenager exerts control over one of the most primary "Maslow" needs – food. Young women, especially, assert themselves absolutely in an attempt to regain control of the self. Well behaved girls don't rebel, get expelled, take drugs or get pregnant – their statement of control is to take back ownership of the most basic need in life – food and drink.

Putting the four pillars together, a sadly typical scenario can be – nowhere near enough of (1) unconditional love – the parents 'don't want to make us big headed'; way too much of (2) discipline; nowhere near enough of (3) encouragement for the same reason as (1) and too much control taken away from the child, rather than (4) allowing the developing human control of their self. (For parents read "parents/primary carers" in case you spent a lot of time with a grandparent or a nanny or elder sibling etc).

Older generations especially seem to have over disciplined their children, set lots of rules, set too many boundaries and not praised their off spring anywhere near enough. The consequences of this are: low self esteem; insecurity; anxiety; feeling worthless; feeling that you don't deserve things; feeling unlovable etc – potentially serious psychological outcomes. As adults we find it difficult to accept compliments because we don't feel worthy of them – we didn't have enough when we were younger to make us realise that we absolutely are worthy of them. Nice comments don't feel 'normal'.

The four pillars (and pillar 0) can provide such a useful model for individuals (and counsellors) to understand quickly and measurably whether there are esteem issues to address and where the roots of these esteem issues may be. Doing this helps the individual to understand that their parenting was not good and it helps them to understand a bit about 'why' this may have been the case, at the outset. This is not about blame, or forgiveness, but about understanding what actually did happen in the formative years and how this may be impacting anxiety, depression, emotions and emotional eating today.

When we know why we are the way we are, we can start to be the person we want to be.

Childhood messages about food

In relation to food, it is fascinating to note the messages that we give children and, therefore, the messages that they carry with them throughout life:

- We tell them to eat everything on their plates. This means we are telling them to ignore their own hunger mechanism (which actually works pretty well in children) and to eat whatever *we* have decided to put on their plate.

- We rarely ask them what they want to eat – we decide instead what *we* think they should have and then battle with them to get them to eat it.

- We try to take away the real enjoyment of meal times for children and insist that they behave and don't play with food. Playing with food is quite natural and can be immense fun.

- We tell them not to talk with their mouths full and yet they want to both talk and eat so this causes a conflict.

- We set meal times to suit our busy lives rather than accommodating when children are hungry and when they want to eat.

- We tell them off for spilling things and yet they don't do this deliberately and they wish, as much as we do, that it hadn't happened.

- We give food constantly as a reward or to cheer children up (they fall over and we give them sweets, they cry and we give them a cookie). This builds up a lifelong connection between eating and feeling better.

We give children all sorts of messages about food that stay with them for life. Look at your own childhood and see how many powerful messages that you are hanging onto that you should now choose to get rid of as a grown-up.

My personal experience was very profound and I have had to work hard to get rid of my early conditioning. My parents were brought up in war time with food rationing and, therefore, had strong ideas about eating everything on a plate and eating whatever was put in front of you whether you liked it or not. My most vivid childhood memories are not of fun playmates or great things that I did, but of constant battles with food and grown-ups. I would spend many afternoons at home in the dining room or kitchen not allowed to leave the table until I had eaten what was in front of me – hungry or not and whether I liked it or not. When I didn't eat it (when, not if) it would come out at the next meal and the next meal until it eventually went bad. I never ate anything that I didn't want to (you can take a horse to water but you can't make it drink) but I certainly went through enough battles making sure that I didn't eat.

The same happened at school. I would spend many an afternoon sat in the dining hall with my uneaten food in front of me watching the clock until 3.35pm when school finished and they couldn't keep me any longer. How pointless and cruel was that? My mother was a teacher at the same school so she would also know that I was in the dining hall and would continue to be disappointed with me. How disappointed was I with the grown-ups? I didn't know just how disappointed (or angry) I was until I first sought help for an eating disorder.

I learned all my later anorexic behaviour during this time. I learned how to push food around the plate to make it look like I had eaten more than I had. I learned how to sit next to 'Greedy Graham' at school so that I could give him the things I didn't want to eat when the teachers weren't looking (a great win-win). I even spoiled my favourite dungarees as a child by stuffing white broad beans into the pockets, when my parents weren't looking, rather than eating them. I learned how to do

180

other 'magic' tricks like slipping food into hankies unnoticed and all the other things that anorexics do like professionals. I learned my eating disorders as a child.

My experience of, and research about, eating disorders convinces me that anorexia is founded on two things – control and self-esteem.

When I became anorexic at fifteen, I was taking control of my life away from the control of grown-ups. One of the most fundamental choices we should have as human beings is what goes into our own bodies. As soon as I was 'allowed' to make more choices about what I wanted to eat and when I wanted to eat I took the ultimate control and hardly ate anything. Trying to control our eating is a euphemism for trying to control our lives. The more out of control we feel in our lives, the more out of control our eating gets. To understand and overcome the emotional reasons for eating we need to be well tuned in to the early messages we received, why we eat and what we really are trying to control.

Regarding self esteem, someone who develops an eating disorder, by definition, doesn't feel good about themselves. They do not like or accept themselves as they are. They are trying to be slimmer. From the low self esteem of not feeling happy in one's body comes the role played by anorexia. The anorexic who manages to achieve the ridiculous goals that she has set herself feels elated and this gives her esteem. (Males also suffer eating disorders, but it is not inappropriate to use the female term here). The bulimic who manages to starve for a day feels the same. The less that can be eaten and the lower the reading on the scales, the higher the self esteem. However, this is not real self esteem based on real achievement. It is a false esteem based on a self imposed target, which is unsustainable. When the starvation inevitably leads to bingeing, the highs of one day become the lows of the next and the distressed individual loses yet more self esteem as they beat themselves up for failing to meet their impossible targets.

Eating disorders don't start off being about food. They start from someone wanting to take control, not having a healthy self image and wanting to weigh less. They become about food, but to overcome overeating we need to understand the underlying emotions.

For any adults reading this, who want to do the best for children, the advice I would offer is to let children do what they want as far as is possible. Clearly they need to eat breakfast by a certain time, but they can choose whether to eat before or after they get dressed, for example, and they can choose what they want to eat. This doesn't mean giving them a limitless choice, as this is equally stressful for children, but it does mean giving them more than one choice (which is actually no choice). You can ask them if they want cereal, fruit, yoghurt, eggs, brown toast or a combination of any of those. Better still, from about the age of five, you can put options on the table and the children can help themselves. (The best way to get a picky eater to eat more is to put the food in the middle of the table and then they think it is scarce and they need to compete for it. They soon pile their plates up and eat quickly).

When there isn't time pressure, ask them when they want to eat (children will generally tell you when they are hungry) and again give them a few options – pasta, chicken and potatoes, ham and cheese – what do you fancy? Then make meal times as enjoyable as possible. Eat with them. Make it OK to spill things. Make it OK to talk. Make it OK to play, within reason. And, whatever else you do, never insist that they eat everything on their plate and never, ever, keep bringing it back again at the following mealtimes until they do eat it. Hopefully this is a pattern of behaviour from a past generation that parents of today are not still following.

I can hear parents now saying 'this is all very well but how do you get children to eat healthy food'? My suggestion is to only make healthy food available and let children play with it. We have had deli bars at home, since the children were aged five and seven, where we put all kinds of things on the breakfast bar and they make their own meals. They have whole-wheat bread rolls, oat biscuits, a huge variety of cheese, cold meats, tinned fish, grapes, tomatoes, fruit and anything else we have in the fridge. They then make their own mustard and beef sandwiches with grapes inside, or cheese, ham and tomato falling out of the roll because there is so much filling. They have a great time and they eat a lot and they enjoy it. It also takes less time in the long run to get all the packets out of the fridge and put them on the table and to get everyone to prepare their own food than it does for you to prepare it and then try to get them to eat what you have prepared.

Why do we see sweets as treats?

It is often said that we have no chance of getting healthy eating messages across to people because the 'food' industry is delivering tens of messages every day for each one that we try to get out. (Notwithstanding the fact that most official 'healthy eating' messages are supporting the 'food' industry!) The same has happened over time with us and sweets being seen as treats. I'm going to start by listing a number of connections between sweet things and emotions and I invite you to add to this list with your own experiences over your entire life. The idea being that – if you can see how often you have had 'sweets equals treats' reinforced over your lifetime, you may realise how many times you need to come up with a counter message and how often you need to tell yourself this counter message to overcome the brainwashing.

-   The doctor gives you an injection and you get a sugar cube 'to take the pain away' (polio is actually administered in a sugar cube).
-   You fall over and get a 'there, there' and something sweet 'to make you feel better'.
-   Every festivity is about food – chocolate eggs at Easter, sweets for your birthday, birthday cake, selection boxes at Christmas, pumpkin pies at Thanksgiving, trick or treat at Halloween and so on.
-   Parties are based around sweets – pass the parcel had sweets in the wrapping, most game winners would be given sweets.

- Tea & biscuits is synonymous with tea & sympathy – cheering us up in some way.
- We hear the sound of the ice cream van and we immediately want an ice cream.
- Holidays bring up many food memories for me – normally 'not allowed' ice cream, we would have a 'knickerbocker glory' in a cafe, we would get sticks of rock at the seaside, we would be eating out lots etc.
- When we went to my grandparents we would always pick up fish 'n chips en route and some 'black pop' and I can remember the whole scenario vividly...

Please add your own recollections because I think that it will help you to see just how many years of conditioning have built up, such that our heads are making a strong link between sweets equals fun equals nice equals good equals I deserve them and all the nonsense that we need to break.

I met a TV producer who gives her son the option of one bad thing a day – crisps, confectionery or a drink – he is growing up knowing these are bad things, not treats. We need to do the same. The park needs to be the treat – not the ice cream van. Buckets and spades need to be the memory from the seaside – not the candy floss.

Breaking the connection

In his brilliant book, *The Power of Now,* Ekhart Tolle talks about 'becoming the watcher'. The first step to breaking negative thought patterns is to be aware that you are having them. You can't stop something unless you bring it into your conscious mind (this is why they say the first step to breaking alcoholism is standing up and admitting that you are an alcoholic). The more connections that you can write down, get out into the open, recognise for what they are – the better you will be able to help yourself. Then you need to become the watcher and be really alert to every time that a voice comes into your head and see it for what it is. You're out on a day trip with the family, you see an ice cream van – make the connection with the associations that this has for you, but then don't blindly go and seek the 'hit' – we will come on to counter messages and strategies next.

If you really do still feel addicted to something or some things – I cannot recommend highly enough keeping a detailed food diary for a while. Within days, you will spot patterns between times of day, where you were, what you were doing and what particularly was 'talking to you' and then you need to take counter remedies to break the pattern that you observe.

When my mother gave up smoking she used this technique to great effect. She kept a diary for a month before and noticed every time she smoked – why, where she was, what she was doing. She then changed her daily routine to avoid the trigger times. She was a teacher and no longer went to the staff room at morning break, as she smoked there. She stopped drinking coffee for a period of time, as she wanted to smoke with her coffee. She wanted a cigarette when she got home from school and actually had a glass of wine instead – twenty years ago that was definitely the lesser of two evils and probably still is.

If you notice that you want a muffin with a cappuccino – either don't go to coffee shops for a while or have a herbal tea – break the pattern that connects one thing with the other. If you reach for something coming in from work – have some crudités ready in the fridge and make sure that you have a good lunch so that you don't get hungry.

The four mind levels

You may have come across this tool in coaching sessions about changing habits – we operate at four levels when we do and think things. The lowest level is unconscious incompetence – we are not aware that we are doing the wrong things. The next level is conscious incompetence – we are still doing the wrong things, but we now know that we are doing the wrong things – we have become the watcher. The third level is conscious competence – we start doing the right things, but it is not second nature. We have to be aware of what we are doing at all times. The ultimate level that we are striving for is unconscious

185

competence – we do the right things without even having to think about it. It really is second nature.

It is said that we can develop a new habit and break an old one in as few as 21 days. This should, therefore, be the longest time that we need to be consciously competent – working hard at doing the right thing every day. Beyond that we will find ourselves doing things automatically. I have always had an automatic 'no' in my head whenever I have been offered a cigarette. For the past 15 years I have had an automatic 'no' in my head whenever I have been offered a biscuit or a cake. I do not even take a moment to consider whether or not I want such processed junk – I just say no. That's where you need to get to as well – with whatever your current fix/addiction is.

Counter messages

When we are aware of the number of messages that we have taken on board about sweets being seen as treats and over how many years – this alone should really help us realise what we have been up against in our minds. Our unconscious has been incompetently saying yes to junk because we haven't broken the connections that have been so firmly established.

We need counter messages and strategies therefore. I have come up with ten here and please make a note of any others, which you think of, that may work for you.

1) We must come to realise that *not* putting junk in our body is the treat – that's being nice to ourselves. Putting the junk in and having the sugar high and low and the guilt and self-loathing – that is really not nice.

2) Please do read labels (I've had clients say that they don't want to know what's in the junk that they are eating). You must take responsibility for what you put in your body and vow to put nothing in if you don't know what it is or if you know what it is and it's not good for you. There is *nothing* more important than your health (physical, emotional, mental and spiritual). Without this you have nothing, so please vow not to compromise your health again.

3) Because we typically crave carbohydrates – remember – every time you eat a carbohydrate you stop your body burning its own fat. Your body will have to get rid of all the glucose and glycogen before you start burning fat again. Is it really worth sticking even one of the children's sweets in your mouth to turn off fat burning for an unknown period of time?

4) If fear works for you – a woman with a BMI of 35 has 93 times the risk of developing type 2 diabetes[27] (a different study for men concluded that the risk was very similar[28]). A BMI of 35 would be an average height woman (5'4") weighing 14 stone 7 lbs (203lb) – that's not breathtakingly high. Sometimes we may think that it is vain to worry about our weight – it's not vain – it's life preserving. Remember that type 2 diabetes is about insulin resistance and I firmly believe that there are only so many times in a lifetime that we can ask the pancreas to release insulin and then it is just going to give up and say 'enough's enough'. I really manage how often I 'hit' my body with carbs, therefore. I respect my pancreas too much to abuse it with a sweet here and a biscuit there and so on.

5) If you need to know some worrying things about sugar, to put you off eating it, I highly recommend a ground breaking book by Professor John Yudkin.[29] This has been credited by Dr. Robert Lustig as a ground breaking thesis, years ahead of its time. Sugar has no sell by date – if it doesn't decompose outside the body, what is it doing inside the body? Sugar is the only substance that we consume with no nutritional value whatsoever – no essential fats, no protein, no vitamins, no minerals – just pure empty carbohydrate calories. If you want to focus on just one substance to give up – put all your effort into giving up sugar and this alone will ensure that you can't eat the vast majority of processed food and this will have immeasurable benefit on your health and weight.

6) Take care that ingrained calorie counting is not giving you false 'permission' to eat junk. Calorie counters may think that an ice lolly from the ice cream van is only 100 calories – where is the harm in that? A few sweets may only be another 100 calories – surely you can have 2,000 calories and not put on weight? Remember that losing weight is absolutely *not* about calories in and out – it is about fat storage and fat burning. It doesn't matter how many or few calories you sneak in – if you register a carb content – you will raise your blood glucose level, release insulin, store fat and you will turn off your fat burning ability.

7) Be acutely aware of how addictive sugar and processed carbohydrates are – remember the highs (which come with equal and opposite lows). You must think of yourself as a drug addict, a smoker, an alcoholic. All of these addicts are told to avoid their fix one day at a time – you need to do the same with your fix. Phase 3 may vary for different people.

    Having been a serious sugar addict, I find that I can eat 85-90% cocoa content dark chocolate most days and I enjoy it, rather than crave it. I go without it on regular occasions – just to be sure that I can. Just because this works for me sadly doesn't mean that it will work for everyone. If you find that you can't have some bread without craving bread again very quickly – you will need to stay off bread. If you can't have dark chocolate without craving sweets and milk chocolate – you will need to stay off sugar. You actually won't feel deprived for very long because you really do, very quickly, get to the point where you don't miss something. You only then miss it when you get a taste for it and then all the desire comes rushing back.

8) The single most important motivational tip that worked for me was – you have to do this sometime so you may as well start today. Tomorrow never comes – so there's no point putting it off until tomorrow every day. Plus, the longer you put off tackling cravings, the worse they become, so just get on with it and do it now.

I kept these words written on a small card, which I carried in my handbag at all times. Any time I was tempted to give in to longings for processed food, I read the card and reminded myself that I would simply perpetuate my addictions by giving in to them. I had to do this sometime so that time may as well be now.

9) Another one that helped me was – it's just not worth it. The old adage "a moment on the lips – a lifetime on the hips" was the feature of a Swedish study published in August 2010.[30] The researchers observed that fast food binges have long-term effects on weight and wondered whether they might change a person's physiology, making it harder to lose and keep off weight in the future." We can offer another explanation – the fast food eaters would quickly develop a taste for junk food (the 'high') and would also develop Candida, Food Intolerance and Hypoglycaemic blood glucose level swings quickly and would find it very difficult to return to their former way of eating after the experiment. The experiment was a month long – more than 21 days – so the junk food eaters would have set new habits and new bad ways of eating even in this relatively short period of time. They would not know why they were continuing to crave these foods unless they knew what we know.

10) We can maintain weight (Phase 3) having a bit of what we fancy – but even then we can't cheat too much or too often and we should always be choosing the foods closest to real food – crisps with just potatoes and sunflower oil, dark chocolate with cocoa/cocoa butter/vanilla and a bit of sugar. We cannot have our cake and be slim. We can't lose weight having our cake regularly anyway and, if we try to have our cake too often when we are slim – we will regain all too easily. We really do need to make a lifestyle and lifetime commitment to real food and do whatever it takes to see junk for the damaging evil that it is.

I really hope that this gives you a few more tools in the kit bag to resist the urges for the foods that you so desperately want, and need, to avoid. If you can harness anger to good effect – be angry that food manufacturers are doing everything that they can to get you to eat as much of their rubbish as possible. They are advertising to you – overtly and subconsciously; they are working hard to make their products irresistible and moreish. Be very angry about this – not just what they are doing to you – but to our next generation. Be determined not to give them a penny of your hard earned cash – you can then gain health and wealth.

Quick summary of Chapter Thirteen

- The 'blueprint' of an adult is largely formed by the messages received by the child up to the age of seven and likely even earlier.

- The four pillars of childhood are necessary for optimal emotional development of the formative child and thus the adults. These are:

1) Unconditional love and positive reinforcement from our parents and/or primary carers.

2) Discipline – All children need accompanying boundaries to go with this unconditional love.

3) Encouragement and respect from our parents and/or primary carers, during the formative years (and beyond) for our own personal development.

4) Self Control – By this we mean "control of the self", the sense of control for oneself – feeling safe and having one's own space.

- Optimal experiences of the four pillars are sadly rare and self esteem issues are likely as a result.

- Additionally, specific childhood messages about food as treats and rewards have embedded unhelpful associations in the minds of emotional eaters.

- To break the connections we need to move from unconscious incompetence, through conscious incompetence to conscious competence and then, finally, to unconscious competence.

- There are many counter messages that we can use to break the embedded connections between food and reward.

Chapter Fourteen

****

Food, control & families

Introduction

Anecdotes can paint such detailed pictures. In a short, true, story an image can be created in the minds of others, which they may well resonate with. I have on rare occasions told an anecdote about when I got my A-Level results. As anyone who has done these exams will know, the date when the results are announced is known weeks (months probably) in advance. Nowadays, teenagers tend to go to the school to get their results. In my day, most people waited for the envelope to arrive in the post.

My envelope arrived and I opened it and was thrilled. No one else asked what I'd got or showed any interest. The envelope sat on the breakfast bar for almost a week – it probably had to be moved each morning to get to the cornflakes! Finally, I plucked up the courage to ask dad if he was ever going to ask what I got. "What did you get?" he said. "Five A's" I replied. He shrugged his shoulders "Just what we expected".

Recently, I was at a dinner party when an attractive, intelligent and caring woman told the same anecdote – almost word for word. I was pinching myself – almost incredulous – it was just too extraordinary that I was hearing virtually the exact same words coming from the mouth of another person. I couldn't believe that someone had had such a similar experience.

As the conversation developed, the continued parallels were just uncanny – neither of us had felt that we could ever do enough to please our parents – our fathers particularly. Both of us felt that we had been constantly criticised. Both of us developed an eating disorder as teenagers and struggled with food related issue throughout our 20's. Equally interesting was where the similarities ended – the other woman is still being constantly criticised by her parents. I am not.

Transactional Analysis

Andy is my sounding board for just about everything I write, so I asked him about this conversation as we were getting ready for bed that evening. "Why on earth would a parent be so dismissive of a child?" I asked him. "Why would they criticise all the time?"

Andy's reply was quite simple: "Control". I didn't understand what he was saying at first, so I asked him to expand. He explained – criticising someone is a way of telling them that they have got something wrong and, by implication, telling them that the person criticising them is right. If you think you're wrong and someone else is right, you look up to them – you look to them for guidance.

We need to introduce a tool for looking at parent-child relationships at this point. The interactions between parents and their children – and adults – are so well known that it has become an entire field of psychology in itself. It's called "Transactional Analysis".

The founder of Transactional Analysis (TA) was Eric Berne. His ground breaking book, *Games People Play* was first published in the USA in 1964 and in the UK two years later, although he had been working on the concepts for some years before this. The book that I really like, which developed the concept of Transactional Analysis further, is Thomas Harris's best seller *I'm OK – you're OK*.

Transactional Analysis is beautiful in its simplicity – it follows the Dr. Wilder Penfield observation that all events are 'recorded' by the child in their formative years (and beyond) and that these recordings are stored – pretty much like an i-tunes collection. There are, in essence, three types of recording and these help us to understand why people behave as they do and how we may be able to help people to change negative behaviours.

1) The Parent – is a large collection of recordings in the brain of external and imposed events, which happened in the first few years of life. All the messages delivered by parents, carers, anyone in a 'parent' role of authority count in this period. Some messages will be 'good and nurturing' e.g. "I love you", "you are lovely". Some will be 'good and useful' e.g. "don't put your hand in the fire". Some will be 'bad and not very useful' e.g. "don't do that" – this one is a problem if it is not obvious why this thing should not be done and if there are many things that inexplicably should not be done. The worst messages, hopefully rare, will be 'bad and counter nurturing' e.g. "You are a horrid child".

2) The Child – this is the equally large collection of recordings in the brain of internal events (feelings) in response to the parent messages. The seeing, hearing, feeling and understanding going on at the time are what we define as the child. "I feel loved", "I feel unworthy", "I feel scared", "I feel useless", "I feel safe", "I feel content" – all such feelings are stored in the collection.

3) The Adult – "is principally concerned with transforming stimuli into pieces of information, and processing and filing that information on the basis of previous experience." (Berne). Harris proposes that there is evidence (Gesell and Ilg, 1943) that, as young as 10 months, the child is beginning to form an adult script from the 'taught script' of the parent and the 'felt script' of the child.

So, from an incredibly young age, we are continually trying to make sense of messages coming in and how we feel about those messages. Followers of The Harcombe Diet do this continually: we challenge every single thing we read and hear and we are no longer 'trusting children' when it comes to public health advice. We are evidence based adults wanting to know facts and where things come from.

It is the 'adult' within all of us that is going to break any parent-child pattern going on. This is the only way forward as 'grown ups'. We now have the freedom to set (fewer) rules, we have the ability to choose with whom we spend time, we can walk towards things and walk away from things, we can eat what we want – we need to make adult choices.

Remember from Chapter Thirteen, Ekhart Tolle's advice to "become the watcher". Watching what you do and how you behave is the absolute first step to changing what you do and how you behave. It sounds so simple but it's very difficult. When I first came across Tolle, I was astounded to see how many times a day I 'beat myself up' and/or ran over a conversation in my head and criticised myself and/or wished I had done something differently etc. First you notice yourself doing it and then you drop it. Someone asks Tolle in the book – but how do you just drop something that is running round in your head? "How would you drop a hot lump of coal?" he replies.

Let's start just dropping it!

A psychologist once suggested to me that two things needed to happen for children to have a good long term relationship with their parents 1) the 'parent-child' relationship needs to be broken and replaced with 'adult-adult' and 2) the adults need to have something in common, so that there is the foundation for a relationship.

There seems to be little incentive for parents to break the parent-child relationship, understandably, as the paternal instinct will likely always have parents wanting to look after us and thinking that they know best for us. It is usually the child that breaks the parent-child roles – with a teenage rebellion or a marriage that the parent doesn't approve of, but this is still child-like behaviour. The only way that a child can truly break a parent-child relationship is to play the role of adult.

If your response to any behaviour is always 'adult', no one can play 'parent' to your 'child' or 'child' to your 'parent'. What we most often see is parent-child in the usual direction and then the child turning into the parent when their parents become dependent in later life. Sadly, so few adults in families manage to have adult relationships and it's because of the power of those early roles that we have.

Back to Andy's comment about control and the explanation that, if you think you're wrong and someone else is right, you look up to them – you look to them for guidance. This is a classic parent-child 'transaction'. The parent (P) criticises; the child (C) feels inferior and, therefore, continues to feel dependent on the parent.

The most wonderful passage on childhood, which I can recall reading, was written by Kahlil Gibran in *The Prophet* (this book has the most beautiful words on everything from marriage to death and more). Here is one line from Kahlil Gibran's beautiful poem on children:

"You are the bows from which your children as living arrows are sent forth."

The 'perfect' parent will be the strong bow, from which the child flies forward. The imperfect parent doesn't want the arrows to fly at all.

There is some excellent writing on child psychology in a book called *A Secure Base: Parent-Child Attachment and Healthy Human Development* by John Bowlby. This book is about 'secure base theory'. A child needs a secure base from which to explore. If their base is weak and so their core feels threatened in any way, they do not venture far from their base. This suits the over protective parents, but does not suit the optimal development of a young human.

The critical parent isn't about you – it's about them. It's about their insecurities – not yours. The critical parent didn't get their four pillars in childhood. They didn't get their sense of self and sense of self worth. This is why they need you to need them – they are trying to derive a sense of self worth from you.

I have sometimes called myself "dinner party fodder". While I would not receive encouragement or compliments directly, I occasionally overheard 'boasts' about how well I was doing at school or in music or sport. Once I had left home, my parents seemed very interested in my latest job title, any appointments or promotions etc – less interested in how I *felt* and if I was doing anything worthwhile in the world. Do you connect with this concept and recognise that you too may be "dinner party fodder"? Something for parents to boast about, rather than someone to praise directly?

The critical parent likely doesn't even realise what they're doing. They would probably be outwardly defensive and inwardly mortified if you pointed out that they never praised you and were far more likely to say something critical than supportive.

National service

There is something unique about the generation that did National Service in the UK. National Service started in 1939 and ended around 1960 – with the last servers discharged in May 1963. My father did National Service and, like so many in his peer group, he was unable to afford to go to university. As dad was very intelligent and studious, the army funded his engineering studies and he stayed in the army for most of his 20's, progressing up the ranks.

Watch any movie and the armed forces are not based on the principles of the four pillars! There is a complete dominance of discipline and rules (pillar 2) and a complete absence of unconditional love, encouragement and respect and control of the self (pillars 1, 3 and 4). The forces decide when the *adult* gets up, eats, works, runs, trains, studies, shines shoes, kowtows to officers and so on. No sergeant major praised my father – he would have been lucky not to have been screamed at or punished in some way.

So then – barely a couple of years after ten years of military service – my brother and I came along and what is the only 'parenting' style known to men who were in the army? I joke that with a military father and a primary school teacher mother – the midwife should have placed a bet on my anorexia being a dead cert!

197

Military service bred a generation where praise was unknown and criticism was the norm. Is it any wonder that the children of that generation have not been praised and continue to be criticised? Women in their 30's to 60's today can be affected by this (i.e. if they have fathers born in the UK between approximately 1920 and 1940). The women saying "I just can't please my father" – probably have fathers who have no idea how to give praise. I bet that these fathers are so proud of us that we would be truly humbled by their adoration, but theirs was not a generation capable of showing this.

Here's an interesting question – does your father praise your mother? I bet you are not alone in feeling his disapproval. I bet your poor mum is also thinking – what do I have to do to please him? And your siblings, and the people who work for him (or used to, if he's now retired) and so on. Don't take it personally – he's the dysfunctional one and there is an explanation as to why.

The generation born to the military service generation can go one of two ways – younger readers may be grandchildren of people who did military service. Sometimes the off spring of the military service generation continue the parenting style that they observed and repeat the same pattern. I see far more often with my peer group that they go to the other extreme. Many of my friends are doing a great job of praising, encouraging, building esteem and confidence in their children – but are still suffering from their own poor parenting.

From parents to partners

There is another interesting dimension to consider, as we look at relationships. In our adult relationships we tend towards things that we are comfortable with, rather than things that are good for us. As I mentioned at the opening of Chapter Twelve, I was trained in Restorative Justice, while working as a Human Resources director and I was fascinated by the characteristics of successful relationships. Apparently, when we marry, our partner is virtually guaranteed to have many of the attributes of our parents/primary carers. Would you be surprised to know

198

that your partner is highly likely to have the qualities of your parents that you *don't* admire and, if you're lucky, some of their qualities that you *do* admire? Write down some words that describe your parents and some that describe your partner and see how many overlap. Are the words controlling and critical in there by any chance?

Everyone needs at least one person in the world to make them feel worthwhile. The most ideal way for this to happen is for great parents to bring up a child with all the pillars intact and then for that child to have innate confidence and self worth for life. Where this hasn't happened, someone can improve their health and wellbeing no end by finding a partner/friend in adult life who makes them feel great. Women are particularly good at doing this with girlfriends – not always quite so good with boyfriends and husbands!

Just as we joke that men marry their mother – have any female readers married their father? The critical one that they can never please? I hope not, but the odds are that some of you will have.

How *not* to make the same mistake with your children

What we need to do as parents is to give our children the four pillars of childhood as foundations for life and in the right balance. This is much easier said than done, as there is a balance between freedom and boundaries and encouragement and caution. As a general principle, however, you almost can't give enough of pillar 1, unconditional love and pillar 3, encouragement. With pillar 4, control of the self, I would recommend erring on the side of freedom from the outset. Then try to give more control of the self as the child gets older and continually reassess how ready the individual child is for more empowerment. Children develop at different paces and some are more ready to make their own decisions at each stage of childhood than others. The flexible parent will notice and respond to this. The second pillar, discipline, is the most difficult one – getting the right setting of boundaries. As a general guide – have as few rules as are really necessary, but make them absolutely non negotiable. E.g. does it really matter if a child puts their elbows on the table? But make always telling the truth an absolute.

What we also need to take care of is that adults who have not had their basic needs met when younger can look to children to fulfil these needs (most likely unconsciously). Parents may love the unconditional love that they get from their children (especially if they didn't receive the same as a child), but we have to take care not to unwittingly place pressure on our children to fulfil our unmet needs. We need to be that bow for the arrow to spring forth and the parent that loves the adoration of their child may find it more difficult to encourage that flight.

Suggestions for dealing with your parents

This next tool isn't just about parents. We will look at this in the context of parents, but this is equally applicable to any work or other life scenario in which we find ourselves. In any situation, we have three options available to us – and pretty much only three options.

1) We can accept the situation.

2) We can change the situation.

3) We can walk away from the situation.

Imagine that you are not happy at work – you can accept it as best you can and put more energy into things outside work, to minimise the impact of work. You can try to change what you don't like – your hours, your role, your department, your location etc – or you can quit. We often don't realise the full extent of options that we have in any situation. Of course there are implications of quitting one's job, but we can feel empowered simply by remembering that this course of action is open to us. We may have to downsize dramatically at home or retrain to change career or take up a few part time jobs to make ends meet – but we need to know that we can walk away from anything unbearable in life, or life can feel unbearable at times.

These three options apply in your relationship with your parents (again – for parents – read any relationship causing you problems).

1) You can accept that they are the way they are and work on minimising the impact that their behaviour has on you. (This is the school of thought that goes something like – you can't change anyone else, you can only change your response to anyone else).

2) You can try to change your parents' behaviour in some way.

3) You can walk away. There is no law in life that says you need to spend time with your parents. I am not recommending this as a course of action – but – like the feeling that you can quit your job at any time – it is a very liberating thought and definitely one to be aware of, rather than to enact.

Let us explore things that may help you with each of these options. It will be helpful to remember the four levels of conscious and unconscious competence and incompetence at this stage, so here's a quick reminder:

"We operate at four levels when we do and think things. The lowest level is unconscious incompetence – we are not aware that we are doing the wrong things. The next level is conscious incompetence – we are still doing the wrong things, but we now know that we are doing the wrong things – we have become the watcher. The third level is conscious competence – we start doing the right things but it is not second nature – we have to be aware of what we are doing at all times. The ultimate level we are striving for is unconscious competence – we do the right things without even having to think about it. It really is second nature."

1) Accept the situation

You have the choice to completely accept the current situation – all the criticism, all the comments about your parenting style, all the digs – whatever is coming your way. You can just ignore all of it and let it go over your head. Men, I find, are naturally good at this. I envy them. I ask Andy how he can stop dwelling on things whenever he likes and he just says "what's done is done – what's the point?" Oh to be male. Women and an increasing number of males are simply not able to do this.

I suspect that, if you could let the current criticism wash over you and not impact you in any way, you would. We would not have thread after thread in our online club about parents, in-laws, bosses and other people who think that they can play the parent to our child (i.e. criticise us/tell us what to do) if we could quite so easily drop these things.

Even if you can't "just drop it", there are two things that you can start doing straight away. Without trying to make any change in the other person's behaviour you can:

a) Understand what is going on. Understand the impact that National Service has had on your father/boss; understand that your mother and other siblings suffer similarly; understand that people who worked for your father would also have described him as critical; understand that this is not personal; understand that this is about him and not you – his insecurities and not your faults in any way.

Simply understanding things gets most people 80% of the way towards a better place than they were before. There is nothing worse than not understanding something and there is nothing more painful than not understanding ourselves. The biggest breakthroughs in counselling often come when the person discovers why they do something – it can be transformational.

b) Ignore what is going on. You can literally, right now, choose to ignore every nasty comment, every criticism and every snide remark about you, your work performance, your parenting skills, whatever – just ignore it. You will not be able to believe the powerful feeling that this can give you – really quickly. You will be choosing *not* to take on board any comment that is not good for you.

Surround yourself with people who energise you and spend as little time as possible with people who drain you. You can physically reduce the time that you spend with people who drain you (parents and in-laws included). Even more powerful, however, is to know that they cannot hurt you, during any time you do spend with them, because you will not allow it. You are metaphorically holding a hand up in front of your face. Think of Vicky Pollard (Little Britain) and you may smile. You are saying "talk to the hand, 'cos the face isn't listening". You do not need to listen to insults or anything that drains you. You do not need energy destruction like that in your life.

Interestingly – you are heading into scenario (2) as soon as you take this route – like it or not (and you should like what this leads to) – the chances are that you are going to start changing the critic's behaviour. If someone is ignored every time they say something, they soon stop saying it. The person trying to play the parent role won't know what is going on, but they will sense a change and it will puzzle them to the point that they will pay more attention to what they are doing and saying.

Every time someone says something unpleasant, your ignoring strategies can include some, or all, of the following:

- Say nothing (I always recommend this one – never respond to criticism unless you are actively trying to change behaviour as we will see in (2));
- Smile sweetly and/or look completely disinterested;
- Change the subject (this is a form of scenario (3) – walk away);
- Busy yourself doing something else (this is also a form of scenario (3) – walk away).

c) You are now effectively into the territory of treating the person trying to play the parent role like a child – you ignore bad behaviour and reward good behaviour. As you do the ignoring bit, simultaneously seize every opportunity to reward good behaviour. If the person who normally moans continually starts an interesting, positive, conversation – join in enthusiastically. If they share some news about someone you both know and say something nice about that person – tell them what a lovely thing that was to say (notice that critical people criticise friends, neighbours and rarely have a nice comment about anyone?) If a critical parent praises one of your children – praise them in turn sincerely: "Oh that's such a lovely thing to say dad – Paul will be so chuffed". All you have to do is reward good behaviour and ignore bad. Enlist your partner's support if you can – it will have twice the effect.

2) Change the situation

As mentioned above, you will move into the territory of changing your parents'/critic's behaviour as soon as you respond differently to how you have done up until now. As soon as you stop playing the child to their parent, they will notice. They are very unlikely to comment, so don't worry.

Let's go back to the conscious competence stuff now and see what options you have to try more actively to change your parents'/critic's behaviour.

By definition, because the critical parent is *not* aware of what they are doing, they are unconsciously incompetent. To move away from this level, someone *must* first become consciously incompetent and then hopefully consciously competent and then unconsciously competent. You can help your parent(s) to become consciously incompetent and then consciously competent. The first step is to point out what they are doing, so that they become aware of it – conscious. This can be done far more easily than you think with comments – either throw away comments, humorous comments, deliberate comments – whatever you think that you can get away with.

As an example, I noticed in my 20's that one of my mother's methods of control through criticism was for everything I did to be wrong. If I was at work late she said I worked too hard; if I was at home in the evening, she said I should be working harder – I couldn't win (ever felt that?) One day, I pointed this out to her – in a very curious/matter of fact way. I simply said "I can't win with you – if I'm at work you say I should be at home and if I'm at home you say I should be at work – which is it?" My mum is very bright (fortunately) and that's all it took for her to be aware of what she was doing – she became consciously incompetent with one comment. The next time she started making the same comment, she actually stopped herself – she was starting to become consciously competent.

So, one option, therefore, is to make comments to make the criticiser aware of what they are saying and doing, with the hope that this may move them from unconscious incompetence to at least conscious incompetence, if not conscious competence. Start as gently or as boldly as you dare. Try humour – test the water. You have quite a lot to gain.

If you have children, you can appeal to the parent-grandparent in them (while not playing the child yourself). Tell your parents that (as an example) you're trying to develop Paul's reading and would really appreciate their help. Could they read with him and encourage him when he gets words right? Suggest that he's been criticised by a teacher and it's knocked his confidence and support from his grandparents would be so valuable etc. Women are the masters of manipulation (apparently) so use it to good effect to help all three generations.

Another option that you should at least be aware of in scenario (2) – changing their behaviour – is that, if someone attacks, you may need to defend. This is a bold and brave step to take (we'll come on to fear), but you must protect yourself (and children if you have them) at all costs. You have done nothing wrong. You have no right to be attacked. You are entitled to defend and should do so as necessary. You would only need a couple of very calm, very firm, comments along the lines of "please don't say that – I find it hurtful", "I wish you wouldn't criticise him like that – it upsets him." If a parent carries on after such warnings – they deserve whatever happens next.

I liken it to a dog snarling. If my niece, Amelie, sticks her face in our dog, Roxy's, face (having been told not to) Roxy will snarl. If Amelie doesn't back away, Roxy will growl. If Amelie still doesn't back away, Roxy will lunge towards her and snap and it's frightening. Then she learns!

You are responsible for your happiness and wellbeing. Your parents are responsible for theirs. The current conflict is that their sense of self is wrapped up in attacking yours and they don't even realise this. Now that you do – if you can't keep it from harming you, you have to stop it.

With my Human Resources (HR) background, I just want to add a note on bullying at this stage. The Advisory, Conciliation and Arbitration Service (ACAS) is a well known organisation in the UK and I have not found a better definition of bullying than theirs. Bullying is described as an act that undermines, humiliates or intimidates the recipient. It is about how the target feels, not whether the perpetrator intended offence.

You can be undermined at work if given insufficient support and information to do your job; you can be humiliated by being picked on in a meeting and 'shown up' in front of colleagues. You can be intimidated to the point of being too scared to talk to the person who has authority over you – sometimes to the point of feeling sick at the thought of going into work. The same three words - undermine, humiliate and intimidate - can describe any situation of bullying away from the workplace. Bullying can occur at the school gate, in communities, in families - anywhere where people interact.

There are only two real options in this kind of parent-child scenario – you cannot accept this situation, for your health let alone any concomitant comfort eating. You must change the situation or walk away. You need to find the courage to tell the bully that their behaviour is unacceptable, with the help of a good HR manager ideally. If this doesn't change things and many bullies are so ingrained in their behaviour it may not, then you need to walk away. Hopefully you can get a role elsewhere in the same organisation. If this is not possible then your health and wellbeing is too important for you to suffer this ultimate attack on the self and you need to walk away altogether.

3) Walk away

Let's go back to our founding relationship now – that with our parents/primary carers. Some counsellors recommend that adults write a letter to their parents setting out how they feel. If you took this route, it would probably be the most emotional thing you ever did. It might also be the most therapeutic. Most counsellors caution against ever sending the letter. The learning is in what you write and getting it off your chest – usually more so than needing it to be read. If you need it to be read – you need to send the letter – that's your call.

The walk away option to me is *not* about *not* having a relationship with your parents. It's knowing that you don't have to. It's knowing that if the criticism doesn't stop, if they continue to drain the energy (and life) out of you – you can just walk away. That really is incredibly liberating (that goes for any persistent energy-zapper in your life – not just your parents).

Remember – you are responsible for your happiness and wellbeing. Your parents are responsible for theirs. It is not selfish to look after yourself – it's a basic human need. It is not your fault that your parents' sense of wellbeing is wrapped up in you playing the child to their parent. That's selfish. It's about being appropriately assertive. It's about protection – it's quite thought provoking that the people we most often need to protect ourselves from are the people who should have protected us from the start.

We need to cover a couple of other things now before we finally pull all this together and talk about food. Who can talk about food and emotions without talking about... guilt.

Guilt

The Oxford Pocket Dictionary definition of guilt is: "The mental obsession with the idea of having done something wrong." What a great definition that is.

With guilt comes obligation. Your parents want you to feel obligated and they therefore need you to feel guilty (I hope that this is unconscious incompetence – anything else would be quite unforgiveable). They want you to visit, they want you to call, they want you to be the dutiful daughter/son, they want you to respect them (whether they deserve it or not), they want you to look after them when they are older. They want quite a lot from you when you think about it.

Here's another great definition – same dictionary – this time for duty: "Moral obligation; what one ought to do."

Can you see the connection between guilt, feeling dutiful, obligation, your behaviour and expectations of you? Can you also see where your sense of guilt came from? When you were constantly criticised by your parents, you developed "The mental obsession with the idea of having done something wrong" – *guilt*. When you could *not* do enough to please your parents (father especially), you developed "The mental obsession with the idea of having done something wrong" – *guilt*. When nothing you did was ever good enough, you developed "The mental obsession with the idea of having done something wrong" – *guilt*. That's where your sense of guilt comes from.

Love

Love should be unconditional. Humans should love another person because they do – not because they want anything back in return. Did you have *conditional* love as a child? You get this, but only if you do this in return (don't wake us up before 9am and you can have chocolate for breakfast – that was one I remember). Be good and you can stay up (the implication being – I don't *choose* to have you around – ouch!)

Conditional love also leads to guilt because it demands things to be done to receive love. It sets expectations, therefore.

It can make someone feel that they have done wrong, because they were *not* loved just because of who they were. There's that "mental obsession with the idea of having done something wrong" again.

Fear

I know some phenomenal people (male and female for this one – more females than males, but still a lot of males) – company chief executives, board directors, lawyers, seven figure salary city high fliers – who are scared stupid of their parents. I know a female who can take on the country's top barrister and won't tell her mother that she isn't visiting that weekend. One of the brightest men I have ever known has had an eating disorder his entire adult life because he is so entangled in his relationship with his mother that he is incapable of taking the adult responsibility that he must take to overcome his bulimia. He also happens to be one of the richest, most successful, most brilliant men I have ever known. He married to meet his mother's expectations, rather than marry my friend, who was the love of his life!

If you feel any fear of your parents – this has to stop. You can never break the parent-child bond if you fear your parents. There is no fear in an adult-adult relationship. Fear was probably encouraged in the same household where the father did National Service. "Wait till your father comes home" is a classic.

What are you afraid of?

Food

A huge part of me hopes that this chapter changes the lives of a few people and no more. I would love it to be the case that only a couple of people resonate with it and that others are thinking "nope – guilt, conditional love, fear – nothing to do with me". My guess, however, is that this will resonate with many of you.

If this has 'spoken to you' in any way, you will hardly need me to draw all of this together into – what has it all got to do with food? Guilt, love, duty, control, what one ought to be doing – are so wrapped up with food, weight and emotions, that you're probably there already. I'll add a few thoughts just to close anyway...

As one of my psychologist friends said to me – "Food is a medicine of choice." Most adults, in today's stressful world, need a medicine of choice – a prop, something that we turn to for pleasure, to blot out the world for a while, for comfort – for all sorts of reasons. Food is just like alcohol, recreational drugs and cigarettes in this respect – it can meet all of those needs. Food is also far more acceptable as a "medicine of choice." We can't turn up drunk at the school gates, but only a fellow bulimic would spot the puffy face of a food addict who binged the night before. Smoking is now socially unacceptable, but we can have a cake with coffee anywhere. Recreational drugs are quite widely used, but frowned upon by many – and yet no one bats an eyelid if your cupboards are full of confectionery and biscuits – your drugs of choice.

This chapter is about emotions, childhood, esteem, control and how you should have developed as a human being and what has likely been missing instead. Because food is our medicine of choice, we cope with all emotions with food. So, we are criticised – we eat; we feel guilty – we eat; we feel guilty because we ate – we eat; we feel angry – we eat; we feel resentful – we eat.

That's what this chapter is about. Unless we understand where all the emotions that drive us to eat have come from – we can't stop this. It has been about trying to hold a mirror up to possible connections. It has been about trying to make practical suggestions about how to deal with the anger, criticism, resentment and all the emotions that drive us to eat – and the source of those emotions – the people who criticise and try to control and try to build their esteem by knocking ours. There are now two more options, therefore:

1) Substantially reduce these emotions. We will never stop feeling guilty, angry, resentful etc on occasions, but we can massively reduce the number of times that this happens and the intensity of the feeling when it does. If we can follow

some, or many, of the suggestions in this chapter, we can reduce the attacks on our self that cause negative emotions.

2) Break the connection with food and the emotion. This chapter hopefully gives many ideas for getting back to an adult-adult balance with anyone who is trying to play parent to your child. I sincerely hope that you take positive steps to stop people hurting you and taking vital energy from you. Even if you don't, or if you do but you don't get all of the way there, you can still stop yourself from reaching for food when you feel angry. Recognise your medicine of choice for what it is and don't take it.

Feel the pain if necessary – it may not be a bad thing. It may drive you to do more of the suggestions in this chapter because it may make you vow not to be criticised again. Getting no support and then reaching for a biscuit tin for support is not a long term strategy. *Not* reaching for the biscuits, feeling the pain of having been let down and then vowing to do something to *not* feel let down again – that would be huge progress.

For me (1) was easier than (2) – taking steps to stop the criticism was easier than taking the criticism and not reaching for the biscuit tin. For you (2) may be easier. Whatever you choose – please choose one option. No one has a right to make you feel bad to the point that you are bingeing yourself into oblivion. I'll say it again:

You are responsible for your happiness and wellbeing. Your parents are responsible for theirs. The current conflict is that their sense of self is wrapped up in attacking yours and they don't even realise this. Now that you do – if you can't keep it from harming you, you have to stop it.

Good luck!

The in-laws

The other interesting dimension that we often see is in-laws. Marrying someone seems to give *their* parents the right to tell you *and* their 'child' how to eat. As many wives experience – mother-in-law (MIL) especially often continues 'her right' to

211

manage the feeding of her son by telling you how you should be feeding him. I have come across many partners who should be awarded medals for restraint and reasonableness following an encounter with MIL particularly!

Given that our whole philosophy is about going back to the way in which our elders ate, you would think that The Harcombe Diet enthusiasm for real food would be embraced. However, the revised dietary guidelines for Americans came out in 1977 and those for the UK came out in 1983 and people who were in their 20's-50's at these times do appear to have been convinced by the U-Turns that the governments of the time made. The key message that people have taken on board is that fat is bad for us. Conversely this generation also took on board the idea that we should be eating carbs at each meal – cereal for breakfast, sandwiches for lunch, pasta/rice/potatoes with the main meal.

There is only one end in mind here – to *not* allow family members, yours or your partners, to derail your healthy eating commitment. Some tips for achieving this are:

1) Not seeing them, or not seeing them at meal times, or inviting them to you, rather than you going there, so that you can serve what you want.

2) In the likely event that you *can't* avoid situations involving food and you know that the topic is likely to be raised, the three routes open are ignore, attack or defend and I personally would probably choose those in that order.

   a) To ignore is very empowering for you and very infuriating for the other person. As MIL tries to engage you in a "My darling Freddie should be having cereal, not bacon & eggs" kind of conversation, just ignore the comment completely. Smile sweetly if necessary – you never have to be drawn into debate. If asked directly (unlikely) "Did you hear what I said?" you can simply say "Yes". This is the path of least resistance and actually it will feel surprisingly comfortable if you choose this option.

b) To attack does not have to be aggressive – it should come in the form of gentle questioning – always questions to which you know the answer but suspect that they don't. Where do you get the idea that fat is bad? When did you change from knowing that meat, butter and eggs were good for us to thinking that they were bad for us? What is the main fat in meat and eggs? Do you know the nutrition of eggs vs. cereal? Do you know how margarine is made? Do you know why we say five-a-day? Attacks, even gentle ones, make someone defend and, if they're defending, they're no longer attacking you. If they do attack back – you've got the facts and common sense on your side.

c) Defending would be my least preferred option. As soon as you find yourself justifying why you eat the way you do, why you feed your family the way you do etc, you stay on the defensive and are vulnerable to attack. What you put in your body once you are a teenager, if not earlier, is none of anyone else's business. It is completely understandable, therefore, to feel outraged when someone tries to tell you how to eat or how to feed your family. If you want their view, you can ask for it.

The final few thoughts on this one are:

- One of the best bits of advice I was ever given (by a teacher when I was in the sixth form) was "only care about the opinion of those people whom you care about." Hopefully the opinion and support of your partner and family matters and is there. If any family members are as narrow minded as most public health diet advisors, then you cannot value their opinion and therefore it cannot matter to you what they think.
- I do find it quite ironic that our elders therefore rejected the eating advice of their elders, when this change in government dietary advice came about, but they expect us not to reject their advice. (The cheekier amongst you may consider pointing this out!)

- The bottom line is – if you let the family saboteurs get to you, they have won if they destroy your commitment. Don't let them win – make each attack and comment make you more determined than ever to look the picture of health and natural weight when you next see them.

Quick summary of Chapter Fourteen

- Transactional Analysis is a field of psychology describing:
    - The parent – the recordings in the brain of all messages from those in authority;
    - The child – the recordings of how the recipient felt when receiving those messages;
    - The adult – the objective assessment of the 'taught script' of the parent and the 'felt script' of the child.

- There is little incentive for the parent to break the parent-child relationship. The child needs to do this by assuming an adult role. If you play 'the adult' no one can play the parent or child.

- We often gravitate towards what we are comfortable with as adults, rather than what is good for us. We may have replicated childhood relationships (with partners or bosses) in adulthood.

- In any scenario, we can accept the situation, change the situation (where possible) or walk away from the situation.

- Guilt, love, duty, control and food are so inextricably linked. We need to be acutely aware of our connections to ensure that deeply ingrained emotional eating does not sabotage our goals.

Chapter Fifteen

✱✱✱✱✱✱✱✱✱✱✱✱✱✱

It's up to you

The most important chapter in this book (once you are free from addiction)

This is the most important chapter in this book. There is only one person in the world who can make sure that you control your eating and that is you. I sincerely hope that this book helps to show you how but, at the end of the day, it is up to you whether or not you choose to do anything about your eating and your weight.

Food addiction

For as long as you are addicted to food, I firmly believe that you do *not* have a free choice about when and what you eat. For you to overeat, when all you want is to be slim, there must be something more powerful than your determination working against you. That powerful thing, which you have to overcome to regain your freedom to choose, is addiction. The smoker is a slave to cigarettes – they feel they have to smoke, rather than that they are choosing to smoke. The alcoholic feels powerless in the face of alcohol – they feel that they have to drink rather than that they are choosing to drink. At the moment you give into that food craving you are in the same boat. You are having to eat that particular substance rather than making a free choice. If you were making a free choice you would not eat it because you do want so badly to be slim. The fact that at the particular moment that you eat the substance you do want it more than you want to be slim is a fantastic demonstration of just how powerful food addiction is.

The goal of this book is, therefore, to enable you to be free from food addiction. You now know that calorie counting will make you hungry and liable to crave anything just to get some fuel into your tank. You also know that Candida, Food Intolerance and Hypoglycaemia can all give you incredibly powerful food cravings for specific foods or groups of foods. You also know that the good news is that you can free yourself from these intense food cravings in as few as five days. If Candida is a problem for you then it can take a bit longer for food cravings to disappear but, even with Candida, cravings will subside dramatically during the five day kick-start eating plan.

When you follow the advice in this book, you *will* get to the point that you are not craving food in general or specific foods. You *will* be free from food addiction and the overwhelming cravings for food that have been sabotaging your eating goals will be gone. This is when it really will be *up to you*.

At this time, when the addiction has gone, you *will* have a choice. You will not have compulsive cravings and you will be free to choose what you eat and when. At this time you need to exercise your freedom to choose on a regular basis. When you are not compulsively craving chocolate, for example, you will have an opportunity to consume chocolate (at any one of hundreds of thousands of retail outlets across the world). You will be able to make a balanced, level headed choice that you will not feel able to make right now. You will be able to weigh up how much you want the chocolate (note the word 'want' not 'need') and what it will do to you if you do have it.

It's up to you

One of my favourite books is the *Seven Habits of Highly Effective People* by Dr. Stephen Covey. It has sold over 10 million copies world-wide so I am probably not alone in this view. Dr. Covey analysed self-help books over decades of literature for his PhD and came to the conclusion that there were seven key themes that emerged in different formats throughout all the readings. He translated these themes into seven 'habits' and proposed that people who adopted these habits would be highly effective people. (A habit is something we do without thinking. We can have good habits, like cleaning our teeth, or we can have bad habits like biting our nails – both of them we can do, without thinking, on a regular basis).

The first habit in Dr. Covey's work is "be proactive." This doesn't just mean the opposite of "be reactive" – it means much more than this. It means take control of your own decisions and actions proactively so that you are always the one who decides what you do.

If you remember back in Chapter Twelve we looked at our basic emotions and how we eat for emotional reasons. We talked about anger as one of the basic emotions and how often we get angry and then overeat later. The really powerful outcome, which comes when a person truly takes control of their actions, is that they know that they can also control their emotions to a great extent. Have you ever found yourself saying 'so and so made me angry'? The reality is that so and so did something and you *chose* to be angry as your response. Now I can hear you screaming at this book already but just stick with me for a while as the readers currently screaming at this book are those with the most to gain by mastering this concept...

The idea behind "*It's up to you*" is that *you cannot control what happens to you in life but you can control how you respond to it.* Viktor Frankl was a Jewish man who survived the Holocaust despite being in four Nazi concentration camps, including Auschwitz from 1942-1945. He suffered the most appalling conditions imaginable and yet he stayed not just sane but content and at peace with himself throughout. While he realised that his captors had control of his body he refused to let them have control of his mind. He decided that his key freedom was that he could choose how he responded to what was happening around him. He could let it destroy him or he could let it make him a better person. He chose the latter. His book about this experience, *Man's Search for Meaning*, is just one of thirty-two inspirational literary works that he went on to write.

One of the London 2012 Paralympic heroes – Steve Brown, GB wheelchair rugby captain, gave an inspirational interview in a British newspaper during the games. In 2005, at the age of 24, Steve lost his balance on a first-floor balcony and fell 12 feet to the ground below. Since that day Steve has been paralysed from the chest down. He allowed himself a couple of nights where he cried himself to sleep and then decided "you can't choose the cards you're dealt, what you can do is make the best of whatever's in your hand." How truly humbling.

You too cannot control what happens to you in life but you can control how you respond to it. There will be times, hopefully few, when real tragedy touches your life and you will feel unimaginable despair, loss and sadness. You will be a healthier person in the long run if you give in to the natural emotions that you will feel at these dreadful times and cry, scream and do whatever you need to do to let your emotions heal you. Advising you to choose your response to situations is not about turning you into a cold and unfeeling robot. It is, however, about getting you to a level of emotional maturity where you *choose* your responses to situations the vast majority of the time. It is also about understanding the times when you will still get angry or frustrated but knowing why you feel that way and why you have made the *choice* to feel that way.

If you think about that last time when you said 'so and so made me angry' think about what they did and why you chose to be angry. Why did you take that anger pill hoping to make the other person feel ill? What did you feeling angry achieve? Getting in touch with our emotions can tell us so much about our overall wellbeing at any point in time.

When I see someone getting road rage, carving another car up or edging up to the car in front so that another driver can't get in, I always ask myself what stress is happening in their life, at that moment, to make them that way. Be serious, we do not get angry enough to kill another person (road rage has resulted in many deaths in the UK and USA) because they overtook us or because they pulled out in front of us. We may be that angry at our partner, family members, children, boss and so on, but we are not that angry at the complete stranger

218

whose driving has come to our attention. The other car driver *chose* to wait until the very end of the lane merging sign before pulling in front of you; you *chose* to be angry about this. That is inappropriate anger, so you need to understand what is really making you angry in your life and what you can do about it.

Understanding why you are really feeling certain things is key to conquering overeating forever. I know now when I want chocolate because I really fancy the taste at that moment as compared to when I am using it as a comfort blanket for an emotion that I am feeling. Or, more accurately, an emotion that I am trying *not* to feel. We use food in a similar way to how alcoholics use alcohol – we use it to escape and numb the emotions that we don't want to cope with in the world. We feel lonely so we eat to cheer ourselves up. It doesn't cheer us up – it just makes us fat *and* lonely. We feel sad so we eat to cheer ourselves up – we then feel fat *and* sad. Talk to a great friend, or a qualified counsellor if need be, but get to the point where you understand why you eat for emotional reasons. This book will help you take away the physical addiction that makes you overeat but you have to work on the emotional bit too.

One of the most powerful feelings that leads people to overeat is very metaphorical. Many overeaters have described a feeling of emptiness which they try to fill with food. "I go to the fridge" said one of them, "I don't know what I am looking for, but I still end up eating something." You will get to the point with The Harcombe Diet where you don't need or crave that food but, if you are still feeling empty inside, you are missing something in life and you need to find out what it is, *because it is not food.*

Whose life is this?

The most seriously overweight people often look desperately for a magic wand to make them slim. They want a doctor to staple their stomach or give them liposuction or wire their jaw so that they can't eat. What they are really asking for is for someone else to take control of their eating because they can't control it themselves. How tragic is this? If you are one of those people who wants control taken away, please give some thought to the following:

- What happened in your childhood with food and control to have given you the messages that you have now?
- How is anyone other than you going to be able to do this for you?

Even when some people have their stomachs stapled, they have been known to liquidise chocolate so that they can still eat it. Who is this cheating? This is like a naughty child stealing cookies from the jar except that it is much more serious. Grown-ups doing similar things are not cheating anyone other than themselves.

The only person who is going to fix your overeating problem is you. This book will explain the physical reasons why you overeat, what is causing your food cravings and it will give you a way out of the addiction that is controlling your life. This book will help you break free from cravings but thereafter it is up to you. You have to choose to do this. You are the one who has to make the difference. You have one life – please don't waste another day of it overeating. Make today the day that you take control and decide – *it really is up to you.*

Games people play

The final emotional/psychological concept, which we are going to review, is about games that we play. Games that are really not helping our weight loss efforts. We need to take a closer look at the top three games being played and develop some tactics for overcoming them:

1) Black and white thinking/all or nothing mentality – whatever we call it – you know what I mean.

2) Beating ourselves up – women are spectacularly good at this.

3) We still think of some pretty disgusting 'foods', as treats.

Let us have a look at each of these in turn...

1) Black & white thinking

Neuro Linguistic Programming (NLP) is the study of how people think and experience the world. As human beings are so individual and subjective, the outcomes of these studies are models of how people tend to behave. From these models, practitioners of NLP can develop techniques for changing behaviour by changing thoughts and beliefs. Here is why changing thoughts and beliefs can be so key to changing behaviour...

The concept of NLP is that for everything that happens there is a belief that is in your head that determines the outcome. This is easy to remember as **A**ction, **B**elief, **C**onsequence (ABC). Here is an example – if you or I were to come second at the Wimbledon Tennis Championship we would be absolutely over the moon. If Rodger Federer were to come second he would be devastated. What is different? The Action is the same – coming second at Wimbledon – but the Consequence is very different because of the two different Beliefs which come between the Action and the Consequence. Our Belief would be that this would be our life time greatest achievement. Roger Federer's Belief would be that he had failed to come first.

There are so many examples of where two people experience the same Action only to have a completely different Consequence because of their different Beliefs. Two people survive the same disaster – one of them has a breakdown and the other lives the most fulfilling life possible. The first had the Belief system "why me?, how can such a bad thing have happened to me?" The second may think something like "I am so lucky to be alive; I will live each day as if it were a gift."

This has really important applications for slimmers because it is not so much the *Action* that is ruining our diets it is our *reaction* to that *Action* – and this is determined by our thought process, our Belief in other words...

As we have explained, there are physical reasons why binges happen. Once you start eating processed carbohydrates your insulin production and blood glucose level go into a roller coaster mode and you will continue to crave processed carbohydrates, to try to elevate your blood glucose level, whenever it drops below normal. You are also feeding Candida which leads to cravings and you are getting your Food Intolerance fix so you will need more of this soon to stop the withdrawal symptoms. Hence there are strong physical reasons why you binge once you start. However, there are also psychological things going on that we need to be aware of – you need to be alert to the sabotage going on in your mind at the onset of a binge…

No one ever ruined a day's eating with that first mouthful. It is what you do after that first mouthful that ruins the day's eating.

- Let us imagine that you have vowed not to eat breakfast and then hunger takes over and you find yourself having a bowl of sugary cereal or,
- You vowed not to eat chocolate and you find yourself buying a confectionery bar as you get a morning newspaper or,
- You vowed to 'be good' all day but then you settle down to watch TV and suddenly those potato chips are calling to you from the kitchen…

Sounds familiar? So you give in to each of the events above but this doesn't ruin the day's eating. It is what we *believe* next that leads to a binge day. What do we say to ourselves? I've blown it today so I might as well eat what I want and then start afresh tomorrow. We can't be 'good' today so we will be 'bad' today and then 'good' tomorrow. And can you recall the relief and excitement you feel once you have made that decision? You suddenly 'allow' yourself to eat whatever you want. You may even get quite excited at the thought of what you will have. I could salivate at the mere thought of chocolate, miles away from getting my hands on it. How Pavlovian is that? (From Pavlov's dogs that were trained to salivate at the ringing of a bell after food was given every time the bell was rung).

But all of this is our mind playing games. Who decided the good vs. bad rules in the first place? You did! Who decided not to have breakfast? (crazy decision) You did! And it was you, again, who decided that the 'good' day was over. You have to be alert to the things going on in your head which are leading you to overeat. Remember – no one ever blew a diet with the first mouthful – it was what they decided to do next (yes decided) that blew it. You never blew a diet with the first mouthful – it was what *you* decided to do next that blew it.

Let's find a few ways around this thinking:

First of all you don't have 'good' days and 'bad' days any more – or rather you don't have them like you used to. A good day now is a day when you are nice to yourself and your body. A good day is when you nourish your body and feed it with vitamins and minerals and nutritious food. A bad day is when you are nasty to yourself and your body. This is any day when you binge or starve, or count calories, or try to give your body less food than it really needs.

Another idea is to introduce the concept of a weight maintenance day. In your old life you may only have had 'good' days or 'bad' days. In your old world these were days when you lost weight or days when you gained weight. Now you can have neutral days, when you neither gain nor lose weight, but you continue to nourish your body and eat mostly healthy food but you have the freedom to cheat. This is exactly what Phase 3 is about. Ideally you will only do Phase 3 when you are at your natural weight but you can have a Phase 3 day at any time.

If you do eat something that you feel you 'shouldn't' have eaten, don't go back to your old style thinking and eat everything except the kitchen sink. Decide to have a Phase 3 day. You won't register lighter on the scales tomorrow but you won't have another couple of pounds to lose that you have just put on today. If you have something you feel you 'shouldn't' then start a weight maintenance/Phase 3 day – don't cheat too much and don't cheat too often. So finish your cheat and then get back on track for the rest of the day. Don't forget to manage the cravings that may come after eating processed carbohydrates and upsetting your blood glucose level. Eat some whole foods to help regulate your blood glucose after eating processed carbohydrates.

Back to our ABC's. Remember it is the *Belief* that leads to the bad Consequence not the Action itself. So let us look at some examples of Beliefs that will lead to different Consequences following the same Action. Let us imagine that you have just started Phase 1 and you find yourself eating a cream cake. There are negative and positive Beliefs that can follow and these can either lead to either a negative or positive Consequence/outcome...

NEGATIVE BELIEFS	POSITIVE BELIEFS
Black & white thinking – I've totally failed. I've got to have no sweet things whatsoever.	Things are never black and white – there is not perfection or failure and nothing in between. Why am I so harsh on myself? Would I treat a friend like this?
Mental filter – I never manage to stick to a diet, I'm useless and I'll never lose weight.	I can lose weight. Others have done it and so can I. It is up to me. There is no outside force making me break my diet. I did really well yesterday and I deserve congratulations.
Blowing things out of proportion – I've blown it now I may as well eat every cake in the supermarket. I'll never look nice for the wedding/party etc.	One cake doesn't mean I've failed. I've just got to get back on track and not let it lead to more than it has to. I can still look nice for the event – no one notices a couple of pounds anyway.

The negative beliefs will lead to you eating every cream cake in the supermarket (and more).

The positive beliefs will lead to you choosing not to let one slip spoil the day and to return to sensible eating straight away.

The key message from NLP or Action/Belief/Consequence is that your Belief, your reaction to something, determines the Consequence/outcome. If you have one slip up on The Harcombe Diet just get straight back on track. Don't beat yourself up. Don't make it worse and don't do any of the following:

- Don't give in to black & white thinking – "it has to be all or nothing so I've failed."
- Don't allow your mental filter to dwell on the negatives and ignore the positives. When you are beating yourself up you are ignoring all the positive things you have done and can do and only concentrating on the negatives. You wouldn't be so nasty to your best friend so don't do the same to yourself.
- Don't blow things out of proportion – "I've had one small slip so it is the end of the eating plan." This is nonsense and you know it. Don't look for excuses to give up.
- My final thought is – you may have noticed that I was privileged to work with some great trainers while I was an HR Director. I remember many of their words of wisdom and here is a great one. It may take a couple of readings, but you'll know when you've got it:

"Whether you think you can or you can't, you're probably right!"

As I mentioned earlier, I kept a little record card in my handbag when I was struggling to give up sugar (I was a massive sugar addict and didn't much care about the delivery tool – biscuits, cakes, ice cream, chocolate, fruit gums – yuck especially the last one). The one thing that I promised myself was that I would read the record card whenever I was wavering. The card changed at different stages of my 'detox' but the single message that always anchored me was – "you have to do this sometime and the conditions and cravings are only going to get worse; so you may as well do it today". The black and white tip that helped me most was – would you treat a pet like this? (I find animals even more 'vulnerable' than humans). The idea that I would starve my beloved moggie and then stuff him with biscuits and sweets and then make him feel bad and starve him again, just appalled me. Then you have to make the connection – why do we do that to ourselves? Then you have to stop it.

2) Beating ourselves up

There will never be a shortage of books to write, but I don't know if I could even start on one that needs to be written – why are women so hard on themselves? We are indescribably brutal to ourselves. (Men – please don't feel left out at this stage – you may well do this to an extent and hopefully you will also find this interesting to better understand the women in your lives).

We are simply 'never enough'. We aren't slim enough. We aren't pretty enough. We aren't a good enough mother. We aren't a good enough housekeeper. We aren't a good enough boss. This is psychological. This isn't about being addicted to biscuits. So, let's float a few ideas about what's going on here. Together we should be able to optimise our understanding of this one.

Working on logical basics – anything psychological has its roots in childhood. The nature-nurture debate is key here and a top book recommendation is Oliver James' quite brilliant *They F*** you up: How to survive family life* (That is the actual title!) If we work on the basis that the one we are most likely to be able to understand is nurture, the four pillars of childhood, from Chapter Thirteen, are going to be very helpful. (You will need to explore nature yourself looking at the characteristics of your parents and your siblings – but I think nurture is going to get us a long way).

I believe that our emotion of never feeling good enough comes from deficiency in some, or all of the four pillars of

226

childhood – and likely – from pillar '0', that our parents' own upbringing may have been less than ideal for their personal development. (Depending on our ages, our own parents were impacted by war – my parents were evacuated very young away from their parents – so this is not about blame in any way – but about understanding how less than optimal development can be continued through generations). If we missed any of the four pillars, we are at risk of not having developed emotionally into a healthy adult.

Parents should tell children that they love them several times a day. They should tell the child s/he is wonderful, intelligent, adorable, gorgeous – every great word that they can think of – several times a day. When the child goes to school (aged 3-5) there will be ample opportunity for other children to 'kick them into touch' if they display any signs of being big headed – but the young human needs to feel confident and assured in this scary world and all of that needs to come from the parents and primary carers from the moment they are born. I look around my peers and see them generally doing a very good job (some too low on boundaries maybe), but I have high hopes for the average off spring of my friends.

What we have tended to do instead (particularly generations who are now in their 60's plus) is discipline the child, set loads of rules, set too many boundaries and not praise them anywhere near enough. The consequences of this are: low self esteem; insecurity; anxiety; feeling worthless; feeling that you don't deserve things; feeling unlovable etc – potentially serious psychological outcomes. As adults we find it difficult to accept compliments because we don't feel worthy of them – we didn't have enough when we were younger to make us realise that we absolutely are worthy of them. They don't feel 'normal'.

What we probably did get was sweets and biscuits and this was given as a treat (when we fell over 'there there', at parties, at festive occasions) and we developed an association that sweets were treats and they made us feel good. Our carers should have been making us feel good with words and hugs, not junk food.

There are two paths of response to this sadly too typical scenario: We can feel sorry for ourselves – poor us, we had a less than ideal childhood, our parents/carers were not as good as they needed to be, we have had inadequate emotional development and have additional challenges for life as a result. All of this is true and important and we are perfectly entitled to feel this way. But it doesn't help us to move on. We can, therefore, choose the path that says "we are where we are", nothing that has happened can be changed – what can we do now to make a difference? Here are a few thoughts:

- Be really aware of what was missing in your development and go out of your way to try to make up for this now. If you had too many boundaries and too much discipline – try to set as few boundaries and rules as possible (more on this below). It is a classic psychological 'truism' that people gravitate towards what they are comfortable with, rather than what is good for them. We can, therefore, emerge from a background of few compliments, find compliments hard to take and gravitate towards a partner who doesn't give many. Surround yourself with those lovely people who say lovely things and practise taking a compliment.

- We are all aware that we know people who energise us and people who drain us. Family can be the most extreme examples of both – we have some wonderful family members whom we can't wait to see and we feel so much better for seeing them. However, family can also be one of the most draining aspects of our life. There is a brilliant part in the Oliver James book where he talks about "notice your behaviour when you go back to your parents' home – especially if it's the actual place that you grew up in – and see the role that you play". We go back to being the little sister, the elder brother, the joker, the 'smoothing things over' person – watch it and be amused by it – but don't let it 'get to you' again. Spend as little time as possible with people who drain you and spend as much time as possible with those people whose company you look forward to and whom you feel sad to leave.

- Women now – set fewer rules. One of the biggest reasons we beat ourselves up is that we set completely unrealistic standards. We set ourselves up to fail. The superwoman/person does not exist – they never did. The more bars we set, the more we will criticise ourselves for not doing things.

Here's life in the Harcombe household – Andy and I both work from home. I set myself a completely impossible to-do list at the start of each day and then feel disappointed when I don't achieve it all (I used to well and truly beat myself up, so I've got better). Andy has a "must/intend/like" list – only things he absolutely must do go on that list (pay a bill before incurring a charge, attend a meeting, phone someone back as promised etc). Then he writes down what he intends to do and he achieves most of this and then he has a couple of 'would like to do if I have a cracking day'. Every day Andy does his must list, much of his intend and sometimes some of the like. He always has a sense of achievement. I have learned so much from Andy and every less than emotionally perfect woman (does anyone know an emotionally perfect woman?!) needs an Andy! We also need great friends of both genders to keep us in good shape. But, fundamentally, we can change our thoughts and behaviours and stop setting ourselves up to fail.

- On the rules and standards – just as we need to set fewer for ourselves, we should set fewer for others. Then we don't get stressed by them letting us down either. Another great book *The boys are back in town* (Simon Carr) is about a dad who has lost his wife and suddenly has to bring up their boys and he finds that the fewer rules there are the better. He ends up letting the boys cycle round the living room, because he can't think of a reason why they shouldn't. Think about all the 'rules' that you set for yourself, your partner, your children – these are all the ways in which you can get let down, beat yourself up and feel bad. Take as many of them away as you can. It is indescribably liberating.

-   The final thought on beating ourselves up is to be aware that it goes hand in hand with punishment/reward; feeling non-deserving and then 'rewarding ourselves'; feeling bad and trying to make ourselves feel good. They are yin and yang and there are two ways of dealing with equals and opposites like this – you attack either one and the other follows. To stop starving you need to stop bingeing; to stop bingeing you need to stop starving. To stop rewarding yourself you need to stop feeling bad and beating yourself up. Would you treat your child, pet, or best friend the way you treat yourself? No – then stop it. No debates in your head, no learned behaviour – just stop it!

3) What is a treat?

This brings us nicely to – what is a treat? Even if we struggle to stop the punishment/reward; feeling bad/wanting to be cheered up kind of pattern – where on earth did we get the idea that junk food is a reward? I know – childhood – but we know better now and we have to read the ingredients on the packet of whatever we are just about to eat and then really connect with what we are about to put in our mouths. I used to eat junk like the best of us, but I would not give some of the things I once ate to any human being. Even if I could be bothered to think of a seriously nasty human – would I give them a Weight Watchers® chocolate brownie? I honestly can't think of anyone I dislike that much.

Here's a passage from *The Obesity Epidemic: What caused it? How can we stop it?*

"If you slap your child, be prepared for any person who may witness this to verbally abuse you, or even to call the police. Give your child glucose syrup, sugar, gelatine (derived from the collagen inside animal skin and bones), dextrose, citric acid, flavourings, fruit and plant concentrates, colours (including carmine, which is made from crushed insects), glazing agents (including beeswax), invert sugar syrup and fruit extract and no one will bat an eyelid. That's the ingredients list for (sing along) "Kids and Grown-ups love it so, the happy world of Haribo®". And – the slap is supposed to be a punishment and the sweets are supposed to be a treat. What could such a concoction do to the body of a child? I believe that loving a child (indeed any human being) and giving them a cocktail of sugars bonded together with animal innards are mutually exclusive acts."

Hypnosis, aversion therapy, find out what these ingredients actually are – do whatever it takes to realise that these are anything but treats and you would have to seriously dislike yourself, or someone else, to give them this kind of chemical bomb. Then don't eat them again.

Quick summary of Chapter Fifteen

- It's up to you.

- No one else is going to make you stop overeating. You have to do it. This book will help you understand the physical reasons for food addiction and cravings. This section, on the psychological aspects of overeating, can help you understand your emotional reasons for eating. But, at the end of the day, you are the one who has to use all of this and make it happen.

- You must believe that you can do this because you absolutely can.

- Finally, you must do it now. Candida, Food Intolerance and Hypoglycaemia do not get better. They do not stay at a steady state. Unless treated they get worse. You have to deal with this some time and the longer you leave it the worse it will be, so sort it now.

The two pieces of paper

****

You now know that you overeat when all you want is to be slim because you have addict-like food cravings. You have these cravings because of one thing that you are doing, calorie counting, and because of one, or all, of three conditions that you may have – Candida, Food Intolerance and Hypoglycaemia.

The key to overcoming overeating is to overcome cravings. You have failed so many times before because of these cravings. Stop counting calories; follow the strategies in this book to overcome the three conditions and you can free yourself from food cravings. When you are free from food cravings you will have a choice as to what you eat and when you eat it. Right now you do not have that choice. You are not greedy or weak willed. You are a food addict and you need to go 'cold turkey' on some foods, just as a drug addict needs to go 'cold turkey' on their addictive substance.

You will succeed this time because you now have the power of knowledge. You know why you have failed before – because of the cravings. You know what you have been craving and why. You know all about three conditions, which you may not have heard of before. You know that you have to eliminate the offending foods from your diet and watch the cravings disappear in literally days. You also know not to starve yourself, or to let yourself go hungry, as this is the surest way to fail.

This is the good news. The bad news is that there are now no excuses. You know why you overeat. You know how to stop it. You know that the only person who can control your eating is you. If you really do want to be slim for life then put all the willpower you undoubtedly do have into fighting food cravings. I can promise you two things:

1) It will be worth it. Your health is the most important thing that you have in life – without it you have nothing. You must nurture, nourish and treat your body well rather than starve and stuff it and make yourself ill.

2) It will be easier than you think. You cannot imagine life without certain foods right now because you are addicted to them. In as few as five days, however, you could dramatically reduce that addiction. Every day that you nourish your body and avoid the foods that are harming it is another day nearer the healthy, slim you.

I know how it feels to be where you are now and I know how it feels to be where I am now. I would love every unhappy, overweight, food addict to be happy, slim and healthy and to be able to get on with something infinitely more important than food – life!

Now that you have the knowledge to overcome food cravings; now that you have the insight to realise the emotional connections you have with food; now that you have realised that this really is up to you, what are you going to do next?

On the following pages, I have written out the only two paths open to you. I want you to read each option carefully and choose one and sign on the dotted line to show that you are fully committed to this course of action.

I know that you'll make the right choice.

Very best wishes

Zoë Harcombe

The two pieces of paper

****

Option one

I vow that I am going to eat what I want when I want.

I am craving things right now, so I am going to give in to these cravings. I know that I have these cravings because I have one, two or three of some quite nasty conditions that cause these cravings. Despite knowing why I have these cravings, I am going to feed these cravings and feed the conditions at the same time.

I know that this will make things worse. I know that the more I give in to cravings, the more I will crave food. The conditions will get worse and my cravings will get worse. I know that I will stay trapped in this vicious downwards spiral getting fatter and sicker.

I don't care about weight gain, bloating, depression… I don't mind feeling foggy, feeling hopeless and feeling helpless… I will put up with having no energy all day long for that momentary relief of having my fix.

I am an addict. I am going to pretend that I am not an addict. I know that alcoholics can't have drink in moderation. I am going to kid myself that I am different – that I can have my addictions (bread, biscuits, cakes, confectionery – whatever it may be) in moderation, despite the fact that I have proven to myself every single day that I can't.

I will have my fix and then try to blank out the guilt and self loathing that follows. I'll probably blank it out by having a binge and then I'll have a carb hangover and won't be able to think much anyway. I will feel useless and out of control and I will be out of control – because I'm an addict.

My addiction will do everything that it can to persuade me to stay an addict for just one more day and I will buy into this because that's what addicts do. That's what I want to believe.

I am not going to do anything about my weight or health today – I'll do it tomorrow. I know that tomorrow will be even more difficult, because I will have fed the conditions more and the cravings will have got worse, but I'm going to conveniently forget this for now. In fact I will always forget tomorrow because I just want my fix today.

I will get fatter and sicker every day that I delay this. That's how little regard I have for the most important thing in my life – my health.

Signed by --

Date --

The two pieces of paper

****

Option two

I vow that I am going to eat for health and weight. I commit this minute to eating real food – if nature didn't provide it, I'm not going to eat it.

I now know why I crave food. Maybe I didn't previously, but I now have the power of knowledge. I know about the three conditions that cause cravings. I know about all the other horrible symptoms that they cause. I know how to overcome them and how to keep on top of them so that they don't return. I know that overcoming these conditions and therefore cravings is the secret to losing weight and gaining health.

I know that this will make things better. I know that the more I stand up to cravings, the less I will crave food. The conditions will get better and my cravings will get better. I know that I will feel increasingly liberated in this virtuous upwards spiral getting slimmer and healthier.

I care passionately about my health and not just my weight. I absolutely do not want weight gain, bloating, depression… I loathe feeling foggy, feeling hopeless and feeling helpless… I will not put up with having my energy, weight and health trashed for even one stupid moment of madness.

I am an addict. I am going to remind myself that I'm an addict every time temptation rears its ugly head. I know that alcoholics can't have drink in moderation and nor can I have any of my addictions in moderation. The longer I go without my addictions the more 'second nature' saying no to them will be and I will soon be at the point where they hold no interest for me at all. I know that I simply cannot have things in

236

moderation. I would so much rather be slim and healthy, than try to have these things that make me fat and sick.

I will not give in to my fix – I just won't. I will take one day at a time. If things are really tough I will take one hour at a time. I know that I have the strength to do this and the more strength I show now, the less I will need in the future, as the cravings subside. It will be joyful to NOT have the guilt and self loathing that go with binges. I will feel in control in a healthy way – because that's where I will be.

I am acutely aware that my addiction will do everything that it can to persuade me to stay an addict for just one more day, but, by just knowing that, I can stop it.

My commitment to health and weight starts today – and I mean today – not tomorrow. Tomorrow really does never come. By making this commitment today, tomorrow will be easier and the day after that easier still and I love the idea that I will then be on a positive journey and not a horrible nightmare.

I will get slimmer and healthier starting today. That's my commitment to the most important thing in my life – my health.

Signed by   ---

Date   ---

Glossary

Candida is a yeast that exists in all of us, which is normally controlled by our immune system and by other bacterial flora present in our body. Candida serves no useful purpose in the body and can, therefore, be viewed as a parasite. In many people this yeast causes no harm and lives within them peacefully. The problem starts when Candida gets out of control and makes its presence known.

An **enzyme** is a protein (or protein based molecule) that speeds up a chemical reaction in a living organism. It acts as a catalyst.

Diabetes literally means "*sweet urine*", indicating that sugar is present in the urine. In people who have diabetes the pancreas does not work properly.

- Type I diabetes used to be called "Juvenile diabetes" as it used to only develop in children, adolescents or young adults. However, we are now seeing this type of diabetes developing in middle aged and older people. The onset of type 1 diabetes is generally sudden and serious.

- Type 2 diabetes used to be called "Maturity onset diabetes" because it used to develop later on in life. However, we are now seeing type 2 diabetes develop in young adults and even children. Type 2 diabetes is by far the more common – 90-95% of diabetics have type 2.

Food Intolerance, means having an intolerance to a particular food or foods. By intolerance we mean an adverse reaction – not an extreme life threatening reaction as with food allergy – but any adverse reaction, which causes the person discomfort. Adverse reactions can include anything from gastrointestinal disorders to headaches and reactions which affect the mental state of the person who has consumed the food.

Glucagon is a hormone produced by the pancreas. Glucagon is, in effect, the 'equal and opposite' partner to insulin. These two hormones work in harmony to keep our blood glucose levels within the critical range necessary.

Glucose is the primary fuel needed by the human body.

Glycogen is the form in which the body stores glucose.

Hypoglycaemia is literally a Greek translation from "*hypo*" meaning 'under', "*glykis*" meaning 'sweet' and "*emia*" meaning 'in the blood together'. The three bits all put together mean low blood glucose. It describes the state that someone is in if their blood glucose levels are below normal. It can manifest itself in a number of conditions, as diverse as fainting, irritability, clammy hands and inability to concentrate.

Insulin is a hormone produced by the pancreas. When we eat a carbohydrate our body converts this into glucose and so our blood glucose level rises. This is dangerous for the human body, so the pancreas ensures that insulin is released to convert the excess glucose to glycogen, to return our blood glucose level to normal.

Macronutrients are nutrients that we need in macro (large) quantities. We know the three macronutrients as carbohydrates, fat and protein.

Micronutrients are nutrients that we need in micro (small) quantities. We know micronutrients as vitamins and minerals.

The **pancreas** is an organ in the body located below and behind the stomach. Its main functions are a) to produce the hormones insulin and glucagon and b) to produce digestive enzymes to help digest (break down) the food that we eat.

A **triglyceride** is three (tri means three) fatty acids bonded together by glycerol (glycerol is a sugar, essentially);

Other books by Zoë Harcombe:

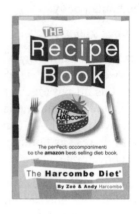

The Harcombe Diet:
The Recipe Book

Real food; great taste; optimal health –
that's what The Harcombe Diet® is all
about and here's how to do it. With over
100 recipes for Phase 1, another 100 for
Phase 2 and some seriously special
Phase 3 cheats, this is the ultimate diet-
recipe book. If you want to eat well, lose
weight and gain health – this is a must
for your kitchen shelf.

ISBN 978-1-907797-07-1

The Harcombe Diet:
Stop Counting Calories &
Start Losing Weight

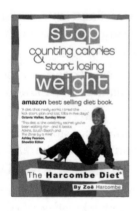

You've tried every diet under the sun.
You've lost weight and put it back on.
The more you diet, the more you crave
food. You've given up hope of being
slim. This book explains why. Count
calories & end up a food addict. Stop
Counting Calories & Start Losing
Weight!

ISBN 978-1-907797-11-8

Copies available on www.theharcombediet.com

Other books by Zoë Harcombe:

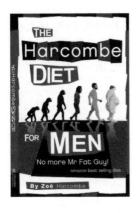

The Harcombe Diet for Men: No More Mr Fat Guy

Men want to lose weight too - fast - and they won't go hungry. They want steak, pasta, cheese and the good things in life, including wine. They'll exercise if they want to; they won't count calories and they want all the answers in just a few pages...
So here it is - The Harcombe Diet® for men!

ISBN 978-1-907797-12-5

The Obesity Epidemic What caused it? How can we stop it?

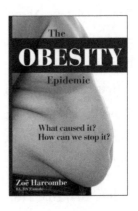

"The Obesity Epidemic is the most comprehensive demolition job on the arrogance and ignorance of the health profession I have ever read". *Barry Groves. Author Trick and Treat: How 'healthy eating' is making us ill.*

ISBN 978-1-907797-00-2

Copies available on www.theharcombediet.com

Index

References

All web references correct at time of going to print

[1] Colleen S.W. Rand and Alex M. C. Macgregor, "Successful weight loss following obesity surgery and the perceived liability of morbid obesity", *International Journal of Obesity*, (1991). (The study results are presented in the summary of this book).

[2] British Dietetic Association's leaflet "*Want to lose weight & keep it off…?*" (http://www.bda.uk.com/foodfacts/Want2LoseWeight.pdf).

[3] Zoe Harcombe, *The Obesity Epidemic: What caused it? How can we stop it?,* Columbus Publishing, (October 2010).

[4] http://nationalobesityforum.org.uk/families/before-you-start-mainmenu-110/34-how-weight-loss-works.html

[5] Dr. Geoffrey Livesey, "The Calorie Delusion: Why food labels are wrong", *New Scientist*, (15 July 2009). Evidence for fat having 8.7 calories per gram.

Max Wishnofsky, "Caloric equivalents of gained or lost weight", *The American Journal of Clinical Nutrition*, (1958). Evidence for fat having 9.5 calories per gram.

[6] Bozenraad, *Deutsche Archives Internal Medicine*, (1911).

[7] Eric Jequier, "Pathways to Obesity", *International Journal of Obesity*, (2002).

[8] Richard Feinman and Eugene Fine, "A calorie is a calorie violates the second law of thermodynamics", *Nutritional Journal*, (2004).

[9] Harris J.A., Benedict F.G., "A biometric study of basal metabolism in man", Carnegie Institute of Washington, Publication no 279, (1919).

[10] http://barrygroves.blogspot.com/2011/10/something-rotten-in-state-of-denmark.html

[11] Francis G. Benedict, *Human Vitality and efficiency under prolonged restricted diet*, (study 1917, published 1919).

[12] Ancel Keys, *The Biology of Human Starvation*, (study 1944-45, report 1950).

[13] Stunkard A. and M. McLaren-Hume, *"The results of treatment for obesity: a review of the literature and report of a series"*, Archives of Internal Medicine, (1959).

[14] Marion J. Franz, Jeffrey J. VanWormer, A. Lauren Crain, Jackie L. Boucher, Trina Histon, William Caplan, Jill Bowman, Nicolas Pronk. "Weight Loss Outcomes: A Systematic Review and Meta-Analysis of Weight Loss Clinical Trials with a Minimum 1-Year Follow-Up", *Journal of the American Dietetic Association*, (2007).

[15] NICE document *Management of obesity: Full Guidance*, December 2006.

[16] http://www.thesundaytimes.co.uk/sto/news/uk_news/Health/article35 9154.ece The Sunday Times 1 August 2010.

[17] http://www.mrc-bsu.cam.ac.uk/BSUsite/CHTMR/AM_forweb.pdf

[18] The Oxford English Dictionary.

[19] "Composition of Foods, Raw, Processed, Prepared, USDA National Nutrient Database for Standard Reference, Release 21". US Department of Agriculture, Human Nutrition Research Centre. (September 2008).

[20] Lieb et al, "The Effects of an Exclusive Long-Continued Meat Diet", *Journal of the American Medical Association*, (July 1926).

[21] Karen Fediuk, "Vitamin C in the Inuit diet: past and present", MA Thesis, School of Dietetics and Human Nutrition, McGill University, (2000).

[22] United States Department of Agriculture nutritional database. www.nutritiondata.com

[23] McIlwain, H. and Bachelard, H.S., *Biochemistry and the Central Nervous System*, Edinburgh: Churchill Livingstone, (1985). Estimates the composition of the brain to be (approximately) 78% water, 10-12% lipids, 8% protein, 2% soluble organic substances, 1% carbohydrate and 1% inorganic salts.

[24] www.idf.org

[25] Montain, S.J., M.K. Hopper, A.R. Coggan, and E.F. Coyle (1991). Exercise metabolism at different time intervals after a meal. J. Appl. Physiol. 70(2):882-888.

[26] http://www.nhs.uk/Livewell/Goodfood/Pages/eatwell-plate.aspx

[27] Colditz G.A., Willet W.C., Rotnitzky A. et al, "Weight gain as a risk factor for clinical diabetes mellitus in women", *Annals of Internal Medicine*, (1995).

[28] Must A., Spadano J., Coakley E.H., Field A.E. et al, "The disease burden associated with overweight and obesity", *Journal of the American Medical Association* (JAMA), (1999).

[29] John Yudkin, *Pure, White and Deadly*, (1972), Relaunched 2012.

[30] Dr. Torbjorn Lindstrom & Asa Ernersson, Linkopings University, Sweden; *Nutrition & Metabolism*, (August 2010)